TABLE OF CONTENTS

Dr. Mark Stengler is a licensed naturopathic medical doctor and a leading authority on the practice of alternative and integrated medicine. An associate clinical professor at the National College of Naturopathic Medicine in Portland, Oregon, Dr. Stengler has served on a medical advisory committee for the Yale University Complementary Medicine Outcomes Research Project and is the author or coauthor of 16 books and the publication, *Bottom Line/Natural Healing with Dr. Mark Stengler.*

TRUE NEW FAT BURNERS NOBODY TOLD YOU ABOUT

THE HORMONE THAT MAY HELP YOU DECREASE BELLY FAT

Sources: **Dennis T. Villareal, MD,** assistant professor, division of geriatrics and nutritional science, Washington University School of Medicine, St. Louis... **Roberta Anding, RD,** clinical dietitian, Texas Children's Hospital, Houston... *Journal of the American Medical Association* .

Researchers say an over-the-counter hormone supplement, dehydroepiandrosterone (DHEA), might help seniors shed stubborn belly fat. Preliminary evidence also suggests that increased levels of this natural hormone secreted by the adrenal gland might help older people avoid diabetes.

THE STUDY...

Belly fat tends to accumulate with aging, just as DHEA levels begin to fall. "DHEA declines progressively with age," explains Dennis T. Villareal, MD, assistant professor of geriatrics and nutritional science at Washington University School of Medicine in St. Louis. "When we're 70 years old, we only have about 20% of the DHEA we had when we were young." From animal studies conducted in their lab, he and co-researcher Dr. John O. Holloszy suspected that falling DHEA levels might encourage weight gain. So in a double-blind trial, they had 56 non-exercising, elderly individuals take either a daily 50 milligram (mg) DHEA supplement or a placebo for six months.

RESULTS...

"The replacement of DHEA, at doses of 50 mg per day, brought back DHEA levels in older persons to the range seen in youth. This resulted in a reduction in abdominal fat that was accompanied by an improvement in insulin action," says Villareal.

Participants taking the hormone supplements lost an average of 6% in visceral abdominal fat—fat deposits lying deep within the abdomen. "It averaged about one kilogram (2.2 pounds) of weight loss per person," Villareal says. Those on the placebo experienced no significant weight loss.

Patients taking the supplements also made significant improvements in insulin activity, lowering their risk for developing diabetes. That's not surprising, according to Villareal, since fatty acids released from abdominal fat cells are known to have a negative affect on insulin action. In terms of health, "what's important is that we saw a specific reduction in abdominal fat, rather than just overall weight loss," he says.

IMPLICATIONS...

Villareal stresses that it's still much too early to recommend DHEA as a weight-loss supplement. "This is only a preliminary study, and we should wait for the results of large-scale, longer studies," he says. "The risks of DHEA haven't been fully defined in this short-term, relatively small study." A larger, five-year trial, involving 176 subjects, is currently under way, he says.

Roberta Anding, a clinical dietitian at Texas Children's Hospital in Houston and a spokeswoman for the American Dietetic Association, calls the findings "exciting," adding that they "open up another avenue for the management of obesity."

However, she says the supplements industry remains largely unregulated. "For the consumer, it's 'buyer beware' out there. I don't know that you can necessarily get high-quality DHEA in every health-food store, that they are all created equal."

She adds that DHEA supplements might be harmful for people with a history of hormone-sensitive cancers, such as tumors of the breast or prostate. Anding says participants in a St. Louis study who took DHEA supplements experienced a "significant" rise in blood levels of estradiol (an estrogen-like hormone) and testosterone, hormones commonly connected to breast and prostate cancers, respectively.

BOTTOM LINE...

Long-term safety data holds the answer to the widespread use of DHEA. "There are going to be some people—individuals with estrogen-sensitive breast cancer or individuals who may have prostate cancer—who really should not take DHEA," Anding says.

■

WHAT DR. MARK STENGLER RECOMMENDS REGARDING DHEA

Hormones are powerful chemicals and DHEA is no exception. It has a powerful effect on thermogenesis, which is the body's burning of calories to produce heat. However, I do not recommend that just anybody supplement DHEA without having their level tested first by a saliva, urine, or blood test. If your levels are low and you supplement DHEA, make sure to have your levels monitored by a doctor every six to twelve months. DHEA also influences testosterone and estrogen levels, and so supplementing too much can imbalance your hormones.

■

DR. STENGLER'S NATURAL ALTERNATIVE TO SUGAR

Artificial sweeteners and the chemical processes used to create them have been making headlines recently. The controversy focuses primarily on the fact that the sugar in Splenda is converted to a sweetener using chlorine. Little information has been published about all the truly natural alternatives to sugar.

The result is that most Americans remain unfamiliar with healthy, natural options like Luo Han Guo, also referred to as Lo Han. A rare fruit found in China, Luo Han yields a powder 250 to 300 times sweeter than sugar.

And that's just the tip of the iceberg when it comes to the benefits of Luo Han.

As a sweetener, Luo Han Guo has no calories, does not elevate blood sugar, and is heat stable—which means it can be added to both hot and cold foods. It also helps prevent cavities and has no after-taste. These attributes make it an ideal, versatile option as a natural sweetener for tea, coffee or other beverages, and for use in making desserts.

ITS ORIGINS...

While Westerners may have much to learn about Luo Han, the fruit has been used in a variety of ways, for thousands of years in China. The Lo Han Guo is a round, green perennial vine fruit in the melon family that grows wild throughout the mountainous terrain of Southwest China. Historic Chinese writings describe Song Dynasty monks brewing the fruit for medicinal beverages more than 800 years ago.

Luo Han, which is typically dried and sold in Chinese medicinal herb shops, has long been used in China and other Asian countries as a food and beverage, and also treats colds, coughs, sore throats, stomach distress, heat stroke, constipation and diarrhea.

The dried fruit is sold in a variety of forms, including whole, liquid, powdered or in a tea.

Often, in Chinese households, Luo Han is cooked with pork as a remedy for lung congestion. In fact, the *Encyclopedia of Traditional Chinese Medicine* recommends 10-15 grams—or one fruit—boiled in water per day, to address lung complaints, as Luo Han is a natural expectorant and helps clear the lungs of airborne pollutants.

The move toward using Luo Han as a sweetening agent is a more recent development.

THE VERSATILITY OF LUO HAN...

In 1995, Procter and Gamble Company patented a process for making a sweetener from the fruit. Now, many sugar substitutes derived from Luo Han are available for manufacturing and home use.

The Luo Han fruit, which is sold mostly in Chinese grocery stores in the United States, can be simmered into a thick, sweet juice and used during food preparation.

There are many benefits to using the Luo Han extract as a sweetening agent and sugar substitute—chief among them is the fact that the fruit contains sweet compounds called glycosides, specifically triterpene glycosides. The body does not break glycosides down like other simple sugars, which means blood glucose or insulin levels do not rise like they do with other sugars—making it ideal for diabetics.

Luo Han also contains high amounts of amino acids, vitamins, minerals, and potent antioxidant properties, which benefit immune function and the body's ability to maintain healthy balance.

DR. STENGLER ON WEIGHT LOSS

Virtually every day in my clinic, patients ask me what I think of the weight loss supplements advertised on infomercials. In my opinion many of these products are not scientifically proven, and they are marketed deceptively.

Prolonged elevation of the stress hormone cortisol can lead to weight gain, especially around the abdomen. Chronic unresolved stress stimulates the overproduction of cortisol by the adrenal glands. As a result blood sugar and insulin levels rise, increasing appetite and fat storage.

Studies have shown that nutritional supplements such as phosphatidylserine (pronounced *FOSS-fuh-TIDE-ill-SEHR-een*) and the herb Ashwagandha can reduce cortisol levels but they should only be used under supervision of a physician. The hormone DHEA can also dramatically bring down cortisol levels.

And we know that exercise, positive mental imagery, deep breathing and prayer are the best long-term methods of maintaining proper cortisol balances. These types of natural approaches have been proven. To read more about them, see page 6.

The articles that follow are from other Bottom Line experts.
They will show you how to put these techniques into practice.

USE YOUR MIND TO HEAL YOUR BODY

Source: **Michael Samuels, MD,** an instructor at San Francisco State Institute of
Holistic Medicine. He has a private practice specializing in guided imagery in
Bolinas, California, and is the author of six alternative healing books, including
Healing with the Mind's Eye. Wiley.

Imagine walking into your doctor's office with high blood
pressure, anxiety or chronic pain from arthritis, and leaving
with a prescription for "guided imagery." You'd probably be
skeptical, but this ancient natural therapy allows you to create
mental pictures that aid healing by reducing stress and improving blood flow throughout the body.

Until recently, many doctors scoffed at this notion.

NOW: Guided imagery has captured the attention of main-
stream medicine as a result of two studies conducted at the
renowned Cleveland Clinic. Researchers there found that people recovering from colon and open-heart surgeries experienced less anxiety and stress, needed half of the typical pain
medication and were released two days earlier when they
used guided-imagery tapes for 15 to 30 minutes twice a day.

To learn more about guided imagery, Bottom Line/Health
spoke with Michael Samuels, MD, who has prescribed the
technique for 25 years as an adjunct to cancer therapy and as
treatment for chronic pain.

Will guided imagery ever gain widespread acceptance?

It is happening already in most hospitals throughout the US.
Guided imagery has been practiced on a limited basis in the US
for about 30 years. Now this technique is gaining popularity as
a result of the Cleveland Clinic studies. Hospitals see the proof
that it works from a practical perspective. It can save millions
of dollars through the early release of patients from hospitals.

It also means less dependence on medication, which liber-
ates sick people from the side effects of drugs. With hospitals
embracing guided imagery, doctors' offices are sure to follow.

What is the physiological mechanism behind guided imagery?

Any illness or surgery creates great stress—even if people are not consciously aware of it. Guided imagery induces a state of relaxation, which releases the stress that aggravates the illness. At the same time, it improves blood flow, which allows a surge of healing antibodies and disease-fighting white blood cells to reach the site of illness.

Guided imagery enhances the immune system as a whole, which defends the body against viruses, bacteria and cancer cells. It can lower blood pressure and heart rate, both of which are useful in preventing and treating heart disease. It can decrease pain and alleviate the side effects of many drugs, including chemotherapy.

Why is guided imagery better than meditation?

Both techniques induce relaxation, but guided imagery uses specific visualizations, which can improve the outcome in people with medical problems.

Are there any psychological benefits?

Guided imagery profoundly affects attitude. It can increase feelings of confidence, control and power, and decrease hopelessness, depression and fear.

What should a person visualize during guided imagery?

You can start by simply putting a picture in your mind. The more realistic the image, the greater your body's response will be.

Picture the place you love best. Relax, close your eyes and fix it in your mind's eye. Add the senses to it. If you visualize the ocean, listen for the sound of the waves, hear the wind whistle in your ears. Feel the soft breeze caress your entire body, the mist brush against your face and the surf splash against your toes. Breathe slowly and deeply. Smell the salt air.

If you have a specific disease, such as cancer, create a mental picture of the disease—a big black blob perhaps—and visualize it being attacked by white blood cells.

Can anyone learn this technique?

Yes. Anyone who has ever daydreamed or can recall fond memories can successfully use guided imagery to help treat physical and emotional problems. Athletes use it all the time. They picture their goal in their mind's eye.

Guided imagery is like learning to ride a bicycle. The first few times you try it, all you can do is think about what you are doing and how you are doing it. Then, all of a sudden, you realize you are doing it with ease without any thought to the process at all.

What tapes are helpful if I want to practice guided imagery on my own?

Two good guided imagery tapes are *Guided Imagery for Stressful Times* by Diane Tusek, RN, president and founder of Guided Imagery, Inc. (440-944-9292, *www.guidedimageryinc. com*) and *Prepare for Surgery, Heal Faster* by Peggy Huddleston (800-726-4173, *www.healfaster.com*).

■

SEVEN EASY STEPS TO GUIDED IMAGERY

Source: **Michael Samuels, MD,** an instructor at San Francisco State Institute of Holistic Medicine. He has a private practice specializing in guided imagery in Bolinas, California, and is the author of six alternative healing books, including most recently *Healing with the Mind's Eye.* Wiley.

For best results, practice this guided-imagery program for 15 to 30 minutes twice a day.

1. *Find a comfortable place where you will not be disturbed.* Sit or lie down with legs uncrossed, arms at your sides or resting on your abdomen. Close your eyes. Inhale slowly and deeply. Let your stomach rise on the inhale and fall on the exhale.

2. *Shift your consciousness to your feet and allow them to relax.* Concentrate on feelings of tingling, warmth and lightness. Next, relax your ankles. Let the feeling continue to the back of your legs and thighs. Let your mind float free. Feel the air moving through your nostrils, and concentrate on the body part you are relaxing.

3. *Relax your pelvic area, abdomen and chest.*

4. *Relax your shoulders.* Spread the feeling to your upper arms, lower arms and hands.

5. *Let your neck relax.* Loosen the big muscles that support the head. Now focus on your head. Relax your scalp, drop your jaw. Soften the muscles around your eyes and forehead.

6. Picture a place you love, such as the ocean or the mountains. Hear, smell and feel this place—the waves crashing, the smell of the fresh air, the mist touching your face. If you have an illness, such as cancer, picture white blood cells eating cancer cells.

7. Stay in this state for the remainder of your session. When you're finished, gently move your feet and count one...two ...three.

■

PROVEN HEALTH BENEFITS OF SPIRITUALITY AND PRAYER

Source: **Marty Sullivan, MD,** associate professor of medicine and director of science and healing, Center for Integrated Medicine at Duke University School of Medicine, Durham, NC.

Marty Sullivan, MD, a leading expert on integrative medicine, talks about the connection between spirituality and health.

In what ways does spirituality make a person healthier?

People with strong spiritual beliefs tend to live longer. They are less likely to develop heart disease, cancer and other serious illnesses. They are more energetic and less likely to feel depressed or anxious.

Some studies have shown spiritual beliefs to be more important for good health than not smoking. That's a striking finding.

How does spirituality reduce stress?

People who pray or meditate experience the relaxation response—a drop in blood pressure, heart rate and levels of stress hormones, such as cortisol.

Prayer and meditation also cause an increase in alpha and theta waves. These electrical impulses in the brain are associated with relaxation.

Even if you do not pray or meditate, having religious or spiritual beliefs can reduce anxiety and increase levels of interleukin-6, a blood protein that indicates good immune function.

One theory is that the social support from spiritual communities—such as churches, meditation groups or yoga classes—helps people buffer the harmful effects of stress.

Of course, people with strong religious feelings believe that God is the healing force.

Not all spiritual beliefs are equally beneficial. People with positive spiritual beliefs—such as the idea that God represents love and forgiveness—do better than those who believe in harsh divine punishment.

Can praying for someone to get well speed his/her recovery?

Many studies have explored the concept of distance healing. One study looked at AIDS patients. Over a period of one year, those who were prayed for were 70% less likely to develop AIDS-related illnesses or other complications than those who were not prayed for.

Is it possible that prayer has a placebo effect—that it works only because people think it will?

In most of the studies, neither the patients nor the doctors knew who was being prayed for. That rules out any placebo effect.

Prayer can even affect the growth of yeast and other laboratory organisms. Obviously, these are not affected by the power of positive thinking.

How can we increase our own spirituality?

Set aside 20 minutes for quiet time daily. Spend it meditating...listening to music...or simply allowing yourself to think about the wonders of nature, a memorable line from a poem, etc.

Read spiritual books, poetry or essays. People who practice formal religion often turn to classic texts, such as the Bible. Others might be interested in reading the works of philosophers or theologians.

Be part of a spiritual community. If you don't attend a church or temple, consider taking meditation or yoga classes...or going on spiritual retreats.

Give to others. Nearly all of the world's religions and spiritual traditions emphasize charitable giving. When you share with others, you form deeper connections with a world that is greater than yourself.

■

TAKING A BREAK GIVES NEW ENERGY

Source: **Timothy B. McCall, MD,** an internist, medical editor of *Yoga Journal* and author of *Examining Your Doctor: A Patient's Guide to Avoiding Harmful Medical Care.* Citadel Press. *www.drmccall.com.*

When your body sends you a signal, it's important to listen to it...or it may start talking "louder." Rather than ignoring the signals, consciously choose to take a break. Sometimes you simply need some time to yourself. Cancel that meeting or workout. Instead, curl up on the couch, and settle down with a bowl of steaming soup and a good book. Afterward, if you feel up to it, light your favorite scented candle, put on some quiet music and practice gentle stretches or yoga poses.

AN EASY YOGA MOVE TO RESTORE BALANCE AND ENERGY...

According to Timothy B. McCall, MD, former scholar in residence at the Kripalu Center for Yoga and Health in Stockbridge, Massachusetts, yoga can be extremely beneficial when stress or illness threatens to overwhelm us, because it restores and energizes at the same time. In the go-go culture we live in, no matter the obstacle, the inclination is to fight through it...but don't. Instead, tune in to what you are feeling inside. Listen and respond to your own body.

MOST IMPORTANT: Don't overdo.

One of Dr. McCall's favorite restorative yoga positions is "legs-up-the-wall." He describes the following pose as ideal to calm the nervous system, ease muscle fatigue and restore health...

• *To begin, find a quiet space* and place a cylindrical yoga bolster or two thick blankets a few inches from a wall.

• *Lie down on the floor,* with your hips elevated on the bolster or blankets, and prop your legs up against the wall so that you are in an "L" position.

• *Adjust your pose to comfort* (closer to or farther from the wall), rest your arms above your head or out to the sides and unclench your hands.

• *Once you are completely comfortable,* close your eyes and exhale. Mentally examine your body from head to toe, slowly and consciously dissolving the tension throughout. Be aware of your breath as it passes in and out of your body.

- *Rest in this position* for as long as you feel comfortable, then slowly open your eyes, straighten up and return to the "real world." According to Dr. McCall, when you surrender to the softness of this pose, you invite any residual knots of tension to dissolve completely, and it refreshes and renews, empties angst and agitation from the soul, and acts as an antidote to exhaustion, illness and weakened immunity.

Whatever route you decide to take to relaxation and renewal, be it yoga, meditation or a cup of hot tea, make sure that you allow yourself the time to take a break. Sometimes it's all you need to accomplish your goals with even more strength and confidence.

■

WHAT I DO TO STAY HEALTHY AND LIVE LONGER

Source: **Terry Grossman, MD,** founder and medical director of Frontier Medical Institute, an internationally renowned antiaging and longevity clinic in Denver. *www.fmiclinic.com.* He is board-certified by the American Board of Anti-Aging Medicine and an assistant professor of family practice at the University of Colorado Health Sciences Center, Denver. His books include *Fantastic Voyage: Live Long Enough to Live Forever* (Rodale), coauthored with Ray Kurzweil, and *The Baby Boomers' Guide to Living Forever* (Hubristic).

We are on the verge of radically extending human life. Within a few decades, a single drop of blood will detect cancer at its earliest stages or reveal preventable diseases that we might otherwise develop later in life. Medicine will be customized, with drugs and therapies that match our genetic makeup. It will be common to maintain a high quality of life into our 90s and 100s.

Our challenge today is to stay healthy so that we can benefit from this revolution. We all know how important it is to watch our weight, cholesterol and blood pressure, but that's not enough. I counsel patients on optimal management of the aging process—and I practice what I preach. **HERE'S WHAT I'M DOING TO INCREASE MY CHANCES OF LIVING LONGER...**

TAKE ADVANTAGE OF GENETIC TESTING...

For about $500 (not covered by insurance), you can get tests that show your predisposition to such conditions as high blood pressure, heart attack, Alzheimer's disease and osteoporosis.

WHAT I DO: I'm almost 60, and genomic testing revealed that I have a gene that gives me a 250% greater risk of Alzheimer's than the general population. The results depressed me for several days, but they motivated me to fine-tune my health. For example, I take supplements* to nourish my brain. I recommend these supplements to most of my patients, but especially those who are at higher risk for Alzheimer's. Always check with your doctor before taking any supplement.

BRAIN NUTRIENTS I TAKE DAILY: 20 milligrams (mg) of vinpocetine (pronounced *vinn-POH-seh-teen*), a nutrient derived from the periwinkle plant that increases blood flow to the brain and has memory-enhancing effects...100 mg of phosphatidylserine, a substance that slows memory loss and is found in the cell membranes of body tissue...500 mg twice a day of acetyl-l-carnitine (pronounced *ah-SEE-til-el-CAR-nih-teen*), an amino acid that boosts brain metabolism...100 mg of ginkgo biloba, a tree leaf popular in Chinese medicine that increases cerebral circulation (ginkgo should be avoided by people on blood thinners, such as aspirin or Coumadin).

To find a doctor or facility that performs genetic testing and offers counseling, contact the American College for Advancement in Medicine, 888-439-6891, *www.acam.org/dr_search.*

GET BODY FAT UNDER 15%...

Some fat tissue is necessary. Fat is the body's primary form of energy and is necessary to cushion vital organs. Too much fat, however, secretes inflammatory chemicals that age your body. Reducing body fat is more important than losing weight.

To determine your percentage of body fat, you can purchase a...

• *Body-fat test caliper,* such as the Accu-Measure Fitness 3000 Personal Body Fat Tester, available for $20 at *www.accumea surefitness.com* or 800-866-2727. This is fairly accurate.

• *Some scales also* measure body fat. They are more accurate than a caliper but also more expensive. See the sculptural

*Supplements mentioned in this article are available at most health-food stores.

glass scale at *www.sharperimage.com* or 800-344-4444 (item #TN425).

WHAT I DO: At six feet tall and 178 pounds, I score very well on all the height/weight charts, but my body fat percentage is 17.9%. I would like to lose eight more pounds to reach my target of 15% body fat.

I keep my carbohydrate intake under 30% of total calories and emphasize fish, lean meats, vegetables, tofu and miso soup. This is similar to the diet of people in the Okinawa region of Japan, which has more 100-year-olds than any place in the world and very little serious disease.

HELPFUL BOOK: *The Okinawa Program: How the World's Longest-Lived People Achieve Everlasting Health—and How You Can Too,* written by Bradley J. Willcox, D. Craig Willcox and Makoto Suzuki (Three Rivers).

INCREASE ALKALINITY...

Our bodies continually produce toxic waste in the form of acid (lactic acid, uric acid and fatty acids), which needs to be removed from the blood or neutralized. Overacidity leads to a variety of diseases.

EXAMPLE: While many people believe that kidney stones are caused by excess calcium, the real culprit is a high level of phosphoric acid, a primary ingredient in carbonated soft drinks.

WHAT I DO: Drink four cups of green tea daily for its alkalinizing effect and antioxidants...and avoid soda.

ELIMINATE SUGAR...

Sweets, fructose, corn syrup and high-glycemic-load carbohydrates (pasta, doughnuts, etc.) are the biggest villains in the aging process. Sugar creates a vicious cycle that wears down the body's cells—it spikes the level of insulin in your blood, which causes an intense craving for even more sugar. I don't recommend artificial sweeteners because of the negative long-term effects.

WHAT I DO: Use stevia, a noncaloric herb that lowers blood sugar and kills the bacteria that cause tooth decay. It has been used in Paraguay for centuries with no health dangers and can be found in health-food stores.

OPTIMIZE TOXIN REMOVAL...

Methylation is a simple biochemical process that the body uses to rid itself of dangerous toxins. Between 10% and 44% of the population has a problem with proper methylation, which can lead to cancer, stroke and other conditions. In a healthy person, methylation neutralizes homocysteine—a toxic by-product that forms after you eat protein. Homocysteine can damage arteries, and high levels are associated with heart attack, Alzheimer's, stroke and cancer.

WHAT I DO: I get tested for homocysteine (the test costs $50 to $100). My level is excellent—below 7.5—but if it should rise, I would lower it with daily supplements, including 50 micrograms (mcg) to 100 mcg of vitamin B-6...100 mcg or more of vitamin B-12...and 800 mcg or more of folic acid. These dosages are much higher than the FDA recommendation, so check with your doctor.

REDUCE INFLAMMATION...

Whenever its equilibrium is disrupted by injury or infection, the body responds with acute inflammation, such as in muscles and tendons. While this acute inflammation usually subsides quickly, "silent" inflammation can smolder in your body for decades without causing any obvious problems.

EXAMPLE: Silent inflammation in the coronary arteries is the reason why many seemingly healthy people suddenly drop dead of heart attacks. People with high inflammation readings suffer more than twice the rate of heart attacks as those with low readings.

WHAT I DO: Take a blood test (less than $50) for high-sensitivity C-reactive protein (CRP). CRP is made in the liver and released into the blood in response to body inflammation. A normal CRP level is under 3, but for optimal health, it should be under 1. To achieve that, I eat at least four servings of fish per week. Fish and shellfish, such as sole, halibut, catfish, cod, flounder, crab, salmon and shrimp, are rich in omega-3 fatty acids and help reduce inflammation. Other foods that decrease inflammation include walnuts, spinach, broccoli, kale and such spices and herbs as turmeric and rosemary. I also take fish oil capsules (2,100 mg of EPA and 1,500 mg of DHA a day).

INVOKE THE RELAXATION RESPONSE...

That's what Harvard Medical School researchers call the meditative state that reduces blood levels of stress hormones, such as cortisol and adrenaline. Long-term exposure to these hormones can lead to osteoporosis, high blood pressure, cataracts and other health problems.

WHAT I DO: I attend an hour-long yoga class three times a week. This lowers my blood pressure and improves my sleep and gastrointestinal functioning.

■

LOSE BELLY FAT AND SAVE YOUR LIFE

Source: Cardiologist **Arthur Agatston, MD**, associate professor of medicine, University of Miami School of Medicine, FL , and consultant, National Institutes of Health Clinical Trials Committee, Bethesda, MD. He is author of *The South Beach Diet.* Rodale. *www.southbeachdiet.com.*

The size of your waist is a better indicator of health risks than your weight. Men whose waists measure more than 40 inches and women whose waists measure more than 35 inches usually have excess visceral fat. Large amounts of visceral fat—which wraps around internal organs, such as the heart—greatly increase your risk of diabetes, heart disease, stroke and cancer.

CARBOHYDRATE CONNECTION...

Diet is the key to reducing visceral fat—specifically, a diet that contains little or no refined carbohydrates.

The carbohydrates that dominate the typical American diet —white bread, pasta, cereal, snack foods, cakes, cookies, candies, etc.—are stripped of fiber during processing. These foods are quickly digested and absorbed as glucose, the form that sugar takes in the bloodstream.

The body must produce ever-increasing amounts of insulin to remove excess glucose and fat from the blood. Elevated levels of insulin promote fat storage in the abdomen.

High insulin levels end up removing too much glucose from the blood. The resulting low blood sugar, also known as *reactive hypoglycemia,* triggers food cravings. The more you give in to the cravings, the more weight you gain.

I have developed a three-phase plan that reduces insulin resistance and food cravings without dramatic calorie reductions. People typically lose eight to 13 pounds in the first two weeks and one to two pounds a week thereafter.

PHASE 1...

For 14 days, eat all the lean meat, chicken, turkey and seafood you want. Eliminate refined carbohydrates—bread, pasta, rice, baked goods, candy and alcohol. These foods have high glycemic indexes. The glycemic index measures the amount by which a specific food raises blood glucose levels.

Eliminating these foods for 14 days reduces cravings for carbohydrates and helps normalize glucose levels. Eventually, you will be able to add some high-glycemic foods back into your diet.

Fruits and root vegetables such as carrots and potatoes also have high glycemic indexes and should be avoided in this phase. You can have as much as you want of other vegetables. To find the glycemic index of various foods, go to *www.telus planet.net/public/dgarneau/health3h.htm.*

You also can have mono- and polyunsaturated fats, such as olive and canola oils. These satisfy appetite, reduce food cravings and help lower levels of harmful triglycerides and LDL cholesterol—key risk factors in people with large stores of visceral fat.

Nuts are also allowed. They are filling and contain mainly monounsaturated fats. Nuts are high in calories, so limit yourself to about 15 almonds or cashews, 30 pistachios or 12 peanuts (technically a legume) daily.

Don't worry about overeating. Eat until you're satisfied—you'll still lose weight. Most of the weight loss that occurs during this phase will come from your midsection.

PHASE 2...

During week three, you can reintroduce refined carbohydrates into your diet. Your body will respond more normally to insulin's effects. You can allow yourself a small serving of bread, pasta, potatoes or rice twice a day. Cookies, cakes, candy, alcohol and snack foods, such as potato chips, should still be avoided.

Continue to focus on foods that have low glycemic indexes. Foods that are rich in fiber, such as brown rice, whole-grain breads, etc., have the lowest glycemic numbers because they are digested slowly and release glucose into the bloodstream gradually.

HELPFUL: Prepare foods whole, or chop them as coarsely as possible. The more work the stomach has to do to digest the food, the more slowly glucose enters the bloodstream. Finely chopped foods—shredded potatoes in hash browns, for example—allow glucose to enter the bloodstream more quickly. Whole fruit is better than juice for the same reason.

OTHER PHASE 2 STRATEGIES...

• *Eat fish at least twice a week.* The omega-3 fatty acids in fish have been shown to reduce heart-attack and stroke risk. Salmon, mackerel and herring are particularly rich in omega-3s.

• *Eat a high-protein breakfast.* Morning protein suppresses food cravings and promotes weight loss. People who skip breakfast experience morning drops in blood glucose that trigger cravings. They also tend to eat more calories during the day. A study of teenagers found that those who ate sugary breakfast cereals consumed 80% more calories over the following five hours than those who ate omelettes.

Try an omelette with cheese or vegetables, such as asparagus or broccoli, or have Canadian bacon, turkey bacon, low-fat cottage cheese or farmer cheese.

• *Snack when you're hungry.* Always try to keep some food in your stomach. It is the best way to prevent sudden food cravings. Rather than grabbing fast foods that are high in glucose-raising carbohydrates, try cheese sticks or a serving of sugar-free yogurt. These foods are ideal because they provide appetite-suppressing protein with very little sugar.

PHASE 3...

This is the maintenance phase of the diet. Once you have reached your desired weight, continue to limit refined carbohydrates to keep food cravings under control, minimize insulin resistance and maintain low levels of visceral fat.

■

2

FALSE CURES AND PROVEN MIRACLES

ACONITE, AN AMAZING HOMEOPATHIC REMEDY

The homeopathic remedy called aconite (pronounced *ah-kuh-night*) (*Aconitum Napellus*) is different from the herb with the same name. Herbal aconite is sometimes used in Chinese medicine in very small amounts. But a homeopathic remedy contains aconite in an almost infinitesimally dilute form—in such tiny amounts, in fact, that many scientists have been baffled by the healing effects of homeopathy.

In brief, the practice of homeopathy is based on the science of "like cures like." For example, a high concentration of aconite would produce results that were just the opposite of what we wanted. One of my colleagues, for instance, took too much of the herb aconite, and was immediately attacked with a number of symptoms that scared the heck out of him—including increased heart rate, elevated blood pressure, sweating, and a feeling of anxiety and of impending doom. We know for a fact that the herb aconite, taken in large doses, is potentially lethal. But in very small concentrations (homeopathic form), it produces symptoms that are precisely the *opposite* of those that my colleague experienced.

That's where "like cures like" comes in—the phrase most commonly used to describe homeopathy. If we know what symptoms are produced by the crude herb, we have guidelines for using the nontoxic homeopathic preparation to cure those symptoms. That is to say, a substance that causes symptoms in a healthy person can be used to cure or improve those same symptoms in someone who is ill.

BEATING THE FLU BUG...

Aconite is one of the most common remedies for an acute, infectious disease like the flu—and I've experienced the results firsthand. I vividly recall one rainy, winter's day in Portland, Oregon, when I felt the symptoms coming on—first the chills, then weakness in my legs, arms, and finally my whole body. Before long, the fever began.

But there was a weird aspect to this start of the flu. I began to have the sensation that something was seriously wrong with my body—and that something terrible was going to happen to me. In other words, the physical sensations were accompanied by mental anxiety along with the onset of a sense of fear.

This was strange. As a trained physician, I was not usually aware of any feelings of fear, even when I became ill. Perhaps this is because I'm generally in good health, and I trusted in my own vitality. **THIS TIME, HOWEVER...**

I wondered what was going on—and mentally ran through the usual checklist. Was my blood sugar low? I had recently eaten, so that didn't seem likely.

Was I stressed out and just experiencing a stress reaction that I'd never had before? That, too, seemed improbable since I wasn't in a particularly stressful situation at that time.

It soon dawned on me that the fear was actually one symptom of the onset of the flu. For this particular combination of symptoms, the most effective cure was likely to be homeopathic aconite.

I knew that if aconite is taken in the first hour of a flu, cold, or other infectious disease, it often stops the illness in its tracks. The first dose had an immediate effect. In less than five minutes, I noticed that I had already started to feel calmer.

I took another dose 30 minutes later. The fever broke. Muscle strength began to return. It was actually a strange experience to feel the sensations of muscle weakness and achiness begin to dissipate within a matter of minutes.

By the end of the day, I was able to continue my regular routine as if nothing had happened. Thanks to the power of homeopathy—and the remedy aconite—I had beaten the flu bug!

CHILDREN'S REMEDY...

Every home should have a homeopathic remedy kit that includes aconite. It's one of the most common remedies to use for many minor childhood afflictions, including ear infections, sore throat, croup, flu, and fever. For example, a homeopathic doctor is sure to recommend aconite for high fever if the fever comes on suddenly; if the child is crying, restless, and anxious; and if one cheek is pale and the other red.

There are two key characteristics of a condition that requires aconite. First, the symptoms usually come on very quickly. If it's a fever, for instance, the onset can occur in just a matter of minutes, and the temperature spikes quickly. The second characteristic is that the illness often comes after an exposure to the wind, especially the cold, dry wind. For instance, if a child gets an ear infection after being outdoors on a windy, cold day, I would recommend a dose or two of aconite within the first 30 to 60 minutes after the symptoms begin. There's a good chance the treatment will abort the whole infection.

I've seen a child who has been screaming in pain from an ear infection become calmer—to the point of falling asleep—within 10 minutes of being given homeopathic aconite. Best of all, the symptoms do not return. It's times like these when you say, "Thank goodness for homeopathy."

DOSAGE: Dissolve two pellets of the 30C potency (strength) in your mouth every 15 minutes for the relief of shock, anxiety, panic attacks, or an acute infection like the flu or ear infection. If there is no relief of symptoms within one hour, discontinue use and use a different treatment.

Since aconite can contribute significantly to the relief of anxiety, it is one of the main remedies for women during labor who feel absolutely certain they are about to die.

NOTE: Dosage is the same for all age groups.

WHAT ARE THE SIDE EFFECTS?: As with any homeopathic medicine, side effects are rarely an issue. By taking aconite too frequently, however, you might bring on symptoms of anxiety. Take enough of the remedy to bring symptoms under control, then reduce the dosage or stop taking it.

■

ASHWAGANDHA—ANCIENT REMEDY FOR STRESS

In the ancient tradition of Ayurvedic medicine—as practiced in India for thousands of years—the herb ashwagandha (*Withania somnifera*) has been used to treat conditions such as fatigue, chronic disease, impotence, and waning memory. Now, in the twenty-first-century United States, this well-respected herb has a new and even brighter reputation as a much-needed stress reliever.

Sometimes referred to as "Indian Ginseng," "Winter Cherry," or "Withania," ashwagandha herb has many similarities to Chinese ginseng. In Ayurvedic medicine, it may be used to treat a number of other diseases besides those already mentioned—including asthma, bronchitis, psoriasis, arthritis, and infertility. Ayurvedic doctors prescribe it in very specific ways that are suited to certain constitutional types. It's often given with the so-called "warming herbs," such as ginger, to increase its tonic effect.

Ashwagandha root differs from Chinese ginseng in having a mild sedative action. This makes it well suited for the Type A person—that is, someone who's always "on the go" at such a high rate that he or she may be headed for burnout.

MULTITONIC...

Research shows that this herb is an excellent adaptogen that helps the body cope with physical and mental stress. Studies show that ashwagandha can help people who have exhaustion from chronic stress, weakened immunity (for instance, if they have cancer), and as a tonic for chronic diseases, especially inflammatory disorders.

This herb also has overall benefits for many body systems. Ashwagandha is unique in acting as a tonic to the nervous system, but also has sedative and antiepileptic effects. It mobilizes different components of the immune system to fight invading microbes and has a modulating or balancing effect if you have inflammation.

A number of animal and laboratory studies have shown this herb has antitumor activity. Ashwagandha has also been shown to have antioxidant activity, so it's helpful in protecting brain cells (which could explain why it helps to prevent memory loss). It also stimulates red blood cell production. Ashwagandha is also said to be a rich source of iron, so it's a potential choice for the treatment of iron-deficiency anemia.

Animal studies have shown that it increases thyroid hormone levels.

Over 35 chemical constituents have been identified, extracted, and isolated in this plant. These include some groups of chemicals such as alkaloids, steroidal lactones, saponins, and withanolides.

Ashwagandha has been used in only a few human studies—far outweighed by the number of animal or test-tube studies that have been done. However, it has remained popular and highly valued through thousands of years of use in Ayurvedic medicine. This is a classic case of an herb that has often been used for successful treatments yet never "proven" by modern scientific research. In my opinion, ashwagandha should be used when indicated. I am sure there will be continued scientific research that will eventually shed light on the reasons why this wonderful plant has proven so helpful to so many people.

DOSAGE: The standard adult dosage is 1,000 to 3,000 milligrams daily of the root.

WHAT ARE THE SIDE EFFECTS?: No side effects or toxicity have been reported with ashwagandha.

Recommendations for…

• *Aging.* For one full year, 3,000 milligrams of purified ashwagandha powder or placebo was given to 101 normal healthy male volunteers, all between the ages of 50 and 59. The herb had some physical effects that slowed the effects of aging for all the men in the study. All men showed significantly increased hemoglobin and red blood cell count. Improvements in nail calcium and cholesterol were also noted. In addition, nearly 72 percent of the men reported improvement in sexual performance.

• *Anemia and slow growth.* Ashwagandha has been shown in two human studies and several animal studies to increase hemoglobin, red blood cell count, and serum iron levels. In a scientific trial that continued for 60 days, 58 healthy children between the ages of 8 and 12 were given milk that was treated with fortified ashwagandha (2,000 milligrams a day). The herb improved the health factors that contribute to growth—leading to a significant increase in hemoglobin and albumin. Researchers concluded that ashwagandha can be a growth promoter in children—and they also noted that these children were less likely to have anemia.

• *Arthritis.* Ashwagandha is used in Ayurvedic herbal formulas for the treatment of arthritis and conditions involving inflammation. In a double-blind, placebo-controlled study, 42 people with osteoarthritis were given a formula containing ashwagandha (along with the herbs boswellia, turmeric, and zinc) for three months. Their health was compared with a control group that received a placebo.

The herbal formula significantly reduced the severity of pain and the degree of disability. There were no significant changes in the control of inflammation, however. For this reason, ashwagandha is mainly used in formulas where inflammation-controlling substances are also part of the mix.

• *Fatigue.* Ashwagandha has been historically used for the treatment of chronic fatigue, especially a patient who shows signs of nervous exhaustion.

• *Memory problems.* Some holistic practitioners recommend ashwagandha for its benefit to the brain. It helps improve the ability to reason and solve problems as well as improve memory. Practitioners of Ayurvedic medicine, who are familiar with these outcomes, often recommend it for patients who are starting to experience memory loss. Studies on rats have shown that it improves cognitive function.

• *Stress.* Ashwagandha appears to help the body cope with the effects of stress more effectively. I am sure that ashwagandha will become as popular as the ginsengs in helping to deal with this all-too-common problem.

■

ECHINACEA—THE BEST-SELLING IMMUNE BOOSTER

It's not unusual to get calls at my office from patients wondering what to do about the cold or flu that just hit them. My first thought is: What natural supplements can they get quickly, right off the shelf?

Well, just about anyone can find echinacea (pronounced *eck-in-ay'-sha*) at a nearby store. It's one of the five top-selling herbs in North America. In fact, it's a worldwide best-seller, as herbalists and doctors in Europe have been prescribing echinacea for decades. Carrying the popular name of purple coneflower (so-called because of its beautiful, purple, daisy-like petals), echinacea is renowned as an herb that enhances the immune system. It's commonly used to treat a number of conditions from flu and the common cold to a range of other infectious diseases.

THE SNAKEBITE CONNECTION...

Native Americans of the Plains are believed to be the first to use echinacea. As today, it was a remedy for colds, coughs, and sore throats, but also toothaches, battle wounds, and even rattlesnake bites.

During the latter part of the 1800s, Plains settlers adopted the purple coneflower as a common remedy; and by the 1920s, echinacea was being sold as a commercial product and prescribed by the many physicians who were comfortable with herbal medicines.

Dr. H.C.F. Meyer of Pawnee, Nebraska, was a keen commercial promoter. Adding his own recommendations to what he had learned from Native Americans, Dr. Meyer sold echinacea as a "cure all" for various ailments. His reputation was considerably enhanced by the claim that he had successfully treated 613 cases of rattlesnake poisoning. **ONE DOCTOR GAVE THE FOLLOWING CANDID ACCOUNT OF DR. MEYER'S OWN, PERSONAL ECHINACEA EXPERIMENT...**

"With the courage of his convictions upon him, he injected the venom of the crotalus (rattlesnake) into the first finger of his left hand; the swelling was rapid and in six hours up to the elbow. At this time he took a dose of the remedy, bathed the part thoroughly, and laid down to pleasant dreams. On awakening in four hours, the pain and swelling were gone."

INFECTION FIGHTER TO THE RESCUE...

I can't say I have had any patients come to me for the natural treatment of rattlesnake bites. (If I did, I would quickly hurry them off to a hospital emergency room for a dose of up-to-date antivenom.) But it's interesting to note that echinacea does have the special property of preventing the spread of infectious substances to tissues.

Echinacea as a healing remedy was introduced to Europe during the 1930s. Since then the preponderance of scientific research on echinacea has been done in Western Europe, especially Germany, where the government plays an active role in funding natural-medicine research. But Canadian and American researchers have recently made similar strides in echinacea research, with clinical studies and biochemical analysis of the healing herb.

Over 400 studies to date have looked at the pharmacology and clinical uses of echinacea. Not all studies have shown efficacy of the herb, but most of the research indicates that echinacea helps reinforce the immune system.

Echinacea is consistently one of the best-selling herbs in North America and Europe. Over 10 million units are sold annually in Germany alone.

Though there are nine species of echinacea, *Echinacea purpurea* and *Echinacea angustifolia* are the two most often used commercially. Most clinical studies are done with these species, especially *purpurea*.

TONGUE-TINGLING CHEMICALS...

Scientists have not reached a consensus about the active ingredients in echinacea. Though researchers acknowledge the herb has many immune-boosting properties as well as anti-inflammatory and antimicrobial effects, they're not sure what chemicals or combination of chemicals are responsible.

It's known, however, that echinacea contains caffeic acid derivatives such as cichoric acid and polysaccharides. The plant also has compounds known as alkylamides that are thought to be important. (Alkylamides are the substances that make your tongue tingle and go numb if you take a hefty dose of straight echinacea.)

Some of these compounds are water-soluble and some are alcohol-soluble. When tinctures, pills, or tablets are being created from echinacea, the manufacturer must go through an elaborate process to extract the compounds. Recent research done at the University of British Columbia in conjunction with the University of Alberta has shown that the ratio of the actives in echinacea is important for optimal immune response. So in other words, not only is it important to have active constituents in echinacea products, but to also have them in a specific ratio or blend.

AROUSING IMMUNE CELLS...

Echinacea doesn't work like the pharmaceutical antibiotics that "kill" microbes like bacteria. Instead, echinacea arouses the immune cells that patrol and defend the body against these invaders. It increases the number and activity of disease-fighting white blood cells, and it activates antiviral chemicals such as interferon. Echinacea can even activate the immune cells that fight tumors. In addition, research has shown that the chemicals in echinacea have the power to inhibit an enzyme released by bacteria, called hyaluronidase. Bacteria normally produce this enzyme to penetrate into human tissue. Echinacea prevents this from happening.

Researchers in a German study found clear evidence that echinacea helps to promote good immune cells, called phagocytes. One group of people were given 30 drops of echinacea three times daily for five days, while people in the control group were given a placebo. The level of phagocytes was measured at the beginning and throughout the study. At day three, the phagocyte activity of those taking echinacea increased by 40 percent. By the fifth day, phagocyte activity had increased 120 percent. When people stopped taking echinacea, immune-cell activity dropped off sharply. After three days, there was no difference in immune-cell activity between the group taking echinacea and the control group.

Leading researchers now feel that echinacea may actually be more of an immune-modulating herb, meaning it has a balancing effect on the immune system. As research continues, this may mean that echinacea may be more valuable than just boosting immune function.

VIRUS SLAYERS...

While there are a host of modern antibiotics for killing bacteria, modern medicine has a limited arsenal of weapons to defeat viral infections. This presents a problem for the many doctors who rely on conventional pharmaceuticals in their medical practice. Over 65 million people in the U.S. each year "catch" the common cold, while another 108 million get the flu—and these are just two of the infectious diseases caused by viruses. Others include genital herpes, which affects an estimated 45 million people, as well as hepatitis C, which afflicts 170 million people in the world. Even a simple viral infection like a viral sore throat poses a challenge for any doctor who relies exclusively on antibiotics and other conventional prescription medications.

Echinacea, like some other immune-enhancing herbs, has a direct antiviral effect. Even better, it seems to summon all the resources of the immune system to help destroy viral invaders.

It also works well in combination with other antiviral plants and herbs. I like to prescribe echinacea in a formula called the "virus cocktail," which is comprised of echinacea, lomatium, astragalus, reishi, and licorice root. The synergistic blend of these herbs tends to be more effective than any one herb by itself.

BACTERIA AND FUNGUS...

Since echinacea enhances the action of your immune cells, it is also effective against bacterial, fungal, and yeast infections. This is especially helpful if you're fighting a bacterial infection, because many bacteria are now resistant to antibiotics (because they're overprescribed by doctors for things like viral infections). If needed, there is no problem using echinacea in combination with antibiotics. As a matter of fact, I find when people are on antibiotics for a bacterial infection and use echinacea simultaneously, they recover more quickly.

At least one study—which included 4,190 patients—confirmed this observation. Researchers divided the patients into two groups and gave about half of them an antibacterial formula that included echinacea (along with two other herbs—thuja and baptisia). Along with that formula, the patients received antibiotics that were chosen by the doctors. For comparison, the rest of the patients received only antibiotics, with no herbal formula.

The results showed the effectiveness of taking herbal antibacterial agents along with antibiotics. In the group that got an echinacea-based formula plus an antibiotic, people were cured significantly faster and there was a lower incidence of recurring infection than in the group of people who just got an antibiotic. Also, the symptoms of "sore throat" and "difficulty in swallowing" were improved much more efficiently in the first group than in the second group.

DOSAGE: Echinacea is generally available as a tincture, capsule, tablet, or cream in the U.S. It's also possible to take it in the form of an injection, though this method is mainly used in Germany.

Glycerine (alcohol-free) tinctures are available. These are good for kids, who especially enjoy the berry-flavored varieties.

• *Tincture*. I recommend 20 to 60 drops of the tincture every two to three hours for acute infections or twice daily for long-term use.

• *Capsule*. I recommend 500 to 1,000 milligrams every two to three hours for acute infections or twice daily for long-term use.

NOTE: High-potency, quality echinacea products are standardized to contain active ingredients such as alkylamides, cichoric acid, and polysaccharides.

Some controversy surrounds the length of time one can use echinacea. Many authors state that echinacea should not be used on a long-term basis. However, there are no studies showing that long-term use is harmful or that echinacea loses its effectiveness.

I generally recommend patients use echinacea for acute infections until they are completely over the illness. For those who are very susceptible to infections, especially during the winter, and do not want to change their lifestyle, echinacea can be used on a long-term basis (although it is not so effective as improving diet, reducing stress, and exercising). Long-term use of echinacea throughout the winter season is common in European countries.

WHAT ARE THE SIDE EFFECTS?: There has been no reported toxicity with echinacea, but two patients of mine have had allergic reactions, with some throat swelling after they started taking echinacea. Such a reaction has the potential of being life-threatening. In both cases, I recommended that my patients avoid using echinacea and switch to other immune-enhancing herbs instead.

There have been some concerns about echinacea affecting fertility. An animal study that appeared in 1999 suggested that echinacea might adversely affect fertility—but, in my view, the research was seriously flawed. Researchers directly exposed hamster eggs to echinacea extract and concluded that at high concentrations echinacea impaired or prevented the sperms' ability to penetrate the eggs.

The flaw of the study is that echinacea is broken down in the digestive system to various components, each of which is highly diluted. Putting echinacea directly on sperm or hamster eggs does not replicate what happens in real life. Perhaps there will be further studies that give us a better idea of echinacea's effects on fertility, but this one isn't worth taking seriously.

Recommendations for...

• *Autoimmune conditions.* There's some controversy about prescribing echinacea to patients who have autoimmune diseases—that is, conditions that become worse when the immune system is overactive. The German Commission E, the government-backed medical board in Germany that helps regulate herbal medicine, recommends that echinacea should not be used in those who have tuberculosis, leukosis, collagenosis, multiple sclerosis, AIDS and HIV, lupus, rheumatoid arthritis, and other autoimmune conditions. The assumption is that echinacea will worsen the hypersensitivity of the immune system, causing a flare-up of problems.

While I often agree with many of the Commission E recommendations, many physicians point out that there have not been any studies showing that echinacea is harmful for autoimmune conditions. I have not seen or read any reports where a patient with one of these conditions was made worse from using echinacea, despite the fact that millions of people take it every year.

That said, echinacea would not be my first choice for a condition like multiple sclerosis, rheumatoid arthritis, or other autoimmune diseases. But when my patients with these conditions have an acute infection, such as a cold or urinary-tract infection, I do recommend echinacea and other immune-enhancing herbs to fight off the infection. Usually these herbs are helpful; in any case, they don't seem to aggravate the autoimmune disease.

Interestingly, German physicians commonly use echinacea as a topical cream to relieve rheumatoid arthritis symptoms. These same doctors also frequently recommend echinacea be taken internally for its natural anti-inflammatory effects. Furthermore, newer research is showing that many autoimmune conditions are due to the immune system reacting to infectious agents, and cross-reacting with the body's own tissue at the same time. In theory, this would make echinacea helpful for these conditions. More studies are needed to tell us exactly what effect—both good or bad—echinacea has for people with inflammatory or autoimmune conditions.

• *Common cold.* I have found that echinacea can help prevent the common cold as well as reduce the symptoms and shorten the duration—but results differ. Some people respond almost miraculously, while others get no benefits at all. Overall, though, echinacea is more effective than over-the-counter medicines, which only help to reduce some of the symptoms of a cold and do nothing to assist the immune system or battle the infection.

One clinical study looked at the effectiveness of *Echinacea purpurea* for 120 patients who had the initial symptoms of the common cold, with "acute, uncomplicated upper airways infection." When these patients took 20 drops of echinacea every two hours for the first day—and thereafter three times daily—they fared much better than another group that took a placebo. At the end of the 10-day study, patients were questioned about the intensity of their illness and the time it took them to improve. In the echinacea group, people averaged four days to recover, while those in the placebo group took an average of eight days to recover.

• *Flu.* Yes, there are a few antiviral drugs that can help treat the flu. However, the clinical data on these drugs does not impress me very much. The most commonly prescribed drug, amantadine, isn't at all effective in the first two or three days.

This is a real drawback because most people experience their worst symptoms during the first 72 hours of a flu attack.

Fortunately, my clinical experience has shown that herbs like echinacea can often help with symptoms the first 24 hours. This is supported by research—but the research also suggests that the size of the dose is an important factor. In a study of 180 men and women between the ages of 18 and 60, researchers compared three different groups. The first group took a placebo. The second got 90 drops of *Echinacea purpurea* every day, which is the equivalent of a 450-milligram dose, while the third group received double that, or 900 milligrams daily. Symptoms of all participants were evaluated after three to four days and again after eight to ten days. The results showed that 90 drops of tincture had little effect, but the people who took 180 drops were significantly better off, with less-severe symptoms that lasted for a shorter time.

• *Skin conditions.* In North America, echinacea has not quite caught on as a topical treatment for skin conditions. But many European makers of skin products are including the herbal ingredient.

A review of 4,958 clinical cases focused on the effectiveness of echinacea ointment. The main researcher in the study concluded that the ointment was highly effective for many skin conditions. These included 1,453 patients with wounds, 900 with varicose ulcers, 629 with eczema, 26 with burns, 222 with herpes simplex, and 212 with inflammatory skin problems. More than 90 percent positive results occurred when the ointment was used to treat burns, wounds, and herpes.

• *Vaginitis.* Reoccurring vaginal yeast infections can be quite troublesome for women. One German study looked at 203 women with this condition. Of the 60 women taking echinacea (while the rest took a placebo or other medicines), only 10 had recurrences of yeast infections.

A BOON IN PREGNANCY...

Pregnant women have to be careful about anything they eat, which includes supplements, so I'm often asked whether echinacea is safe to use during pregnancy. My answer is yes. Echinacea has a long history of use by herbalists and naturopathic doctors for the treatment of acute infections during pregnancy. If a pregnant woman has a cold, flu, or urinary-tract infection, I would not hesitate to recommend echinacea. Side effects or problems with the pregnancy or health of the baby have not been reported. In fact, my wife used echinacea during her entire first pregnancy with no adverse effects.

A study by the Hospital for Sick Children in Toronto, in conjunction with the Canadian Naturopathic College, has confirmed the safety of echinacea use during pregnancy. A group of 206 women who used echinacea during pregnancy for upper-respiratory-tract infections were analyzed along with a control group of 198 pregnant women who had upper-respiratory-tract infections but never used echinacea. The researchers found no association with the use of echinacea and birth defects. There were also no differences in the rate of live births or spontaneous abortions between the two groups.

BENEFITS FOR ATHLETES...

Sports medicine specialists studied the effect of echinacea on men who participated in triathlons—those grueling events that involve long-distance swimming, running, and cycling. It is well known that triathletes are at an increased risk for infection because they train so exhaustively for each event. Among the participants of the study, some took a placebo, others were given a mineral supplement (43 milligrams of magnesium), while a third group took 8 milliliters of *Echinacea purpurea* daily. All three groups of athletes took the supplements for 28 days before a triathlon.

During training, one-quarter to one-third of the athletes taking a placebo or mineral supplement ended up getting colds. (Those taking magnesium missed 13 days of training, while those in the placebo group missed a total of 24 days.) None of those who were taking echinacea showed any cold symptoms, and none missed any training days.

■

GINKGO BILOBA—A POWER PLANT

While ginkgo may well be the most widely publicized herb to come along in the past 50 years, the history of its healing powers certainly predates its current popularity. In fact, the Chinese have known about it and have used it for over 3,500 years.

Ginkgo ranks among the top five herbs that I prescribe to patients on a daily basis. Millions of people around the world use ginkgo every day. In countries such as Germany and France, where doctors are accustomed to writing herbal prescriptions, ginkgo is among the most commonly prescribed medicines. European doctors use it to treat a wide range of conditions—from memory impairment, dizziness, and ringing in the ears (tinnitus) to headaches and depression. There are even more uses—such as a blood mover for improved circulation.

If ginkgo trees could speak for themselves, some would give first-person accounts of Aztecs, Vikings, and the Battle of Hastings, since the grandparents of the species have lived as long as 1,000 years. Some reach a height of 120 feet, with a girth of 48 inches. Apart from longevity, ginkgoes boast venerable ancestors.

Fossil records show that the ginkgo is the world's oldest living species of tree. It's very hardy, able to thrive in extreme heat and cold, and to withstand the sinus-hammering pollution of downtown Los Angeles or New York. It's also almost pest-proof—there doesn't seem to be an insect that can do serious damage to this hardy tree.

The leaves, the source of ginkgo medicinals, are fan-shaped and bilobed, resembling the maidenhair fern. The resemblance is so close, it's sometimes called the "maidenhair tree."

TURNING OVER AN OLD LEAF...

Researchers in the 1950s, having heard of the medicinal powers of ginkgo (tree) leaves, began mashing and distilling the components in search of the so-called active ingredients—that is, the chemical compounds that seemed to have potential healing power. What are believed to be the key medicinal ingredients have now been identified. I know it would be rash to say these are all the active, healing constituents—certainly more will be discovered—but at least we're starting to understand how some of the ginkgo-leaf ingredients make important contributions to improved health.

While the active constituents are important, however, I remind people that it's best to use the whole herb rather than focus on one ingredient or component. Studies have shown, however, that the whole herb plus standardized active constituents are more effective than just using the isolated active constituents.

The two groups of active components include flavone glycosides and terpene lactones. Quality ginkgo products are "standardized" to 24% flavone glycosides and 6% terpene lactones —which is a virtual guarantee that the products contain at least these proportions of those particular ingredients. Such products have the same proportion of these ingredients as the extract that's used in clinical studies.

POTENT CELL PROTECTOR...

Flavone glycosides are types of bioflavonoids, the plant-based compounds that are found in oranges and other fruits and vegetables. With bioflavonoids, ginkgo has been blessed with the potent powers of an antioxidant. That means if you take ginkgo, you're less likely to suffer the cellular damage caused by free radicals—unstable molecules that are a result of metabolic activities in the body and environmental pollution.

Many researchers believe that ginkgo produces more antioxidant activity than many of the better-known vitamin antioxidants such as C, E, and beta carotene. Several studies have demonstrated that ginkgo exerts antioxidant activity in the brain, eyes, and cardiovascular system. This could easily explain why ginkgo seems to be effective in the prevention and treatment of diseases that affect those parts of the body—including Alzheimer's disease, strokes, cataracts, macular degeneration, and diabetic retinopathy.

Ginkgo bioflavonoids also protect blood vessels by strengthening and reducing inflammation of their elastic walls. So that's an additional benefit of this herb—significant in helping to relieve varicose veins and reverse the effects of cardiovascular disease.

KEEPING UP CIRCULATION...

In addition to the bioflavonoids, ginkgo has another component, unique to this plant. A family of terpene lactones, specifically called ginkgolides and bilobalides, give ginkgo an extraordinary ability to increase circulation to the brain and extremities. The substances cause the blood vessel walls to relax and dilate, which permits increased blood flow. They also have what's called a "tonifying effect" on the venous system, allowing for the more efficient return of blood to the heart.

Ginkgo also has a natural blood-thinning effect. It helps to prevent blood platelets from sticking together—and platelets are the cells that form blood clots.

The way ginkgo improves circulation is particularly impressive. In one study where researchers measured the blood flow through capillaries in healthy adults, they found a 57 percent increase in blood flow among those who were regularly taking ginkgo. This finding is particularly important to seniors. As we age, we're more likely to have blockages in the blood flow that reaches the brain and other parts of the bodies. These problems are directly attributable to plaque buildup in the arteries. Ginkgo acts as sort of a bypass mechanism, helping the blood make its way through partially clogged arteries.

NERVE RENEWAL...

The ginkgolides also help protect nerve cells from being damaged. This is important for people who are recovering from a stroke. In addition, some ongoing research will probably show whether ginkgo has the benefits that it's reputed to possess for people who are recovering from brain trauma. What's certain is that nerve cells need the kind of protection that ginkgo provides—particularly people (such as those with diabetes) who have problems with neuropathy (nerve disorder).

DOSAGE: As a standard dosage, I recommend a ginkgo extract standardized to 24% flavone glycosides and 6% terpene lactones. Dosages used in studies range from 120 milligrams to 360 milligrams daily. Most of my patients take 60 milligrams two to four times daily, for a daily total of 120 to 240 milligrams. The vast majority report beneficial results.

For severe cases, like early-stage Alzheimer's disease, I recommend that people take 240 to 360 milligrams daily.

If you start to take ginkgo for a particular condition or for general health, I suggest you continue taking it for at least eight weeks to assess its therapeutic effect. Most of my patients who take it to improve their memory or help their circulation notice the beginnings of improvements within about a month.

Ginkgo supplements are available in capsule, tablet, and tincture form.

WHAT ARE THE SIDE EFFECTS?: Doctors, researchers, and practitioners have noted very few adverse effects among people who take ginkgo. A small number—less than 1 percent of those who take it—have reported mild digestive upset.

Other rare side effects mentioned in the literature include headaches and dizziness. I've had very few patients who complained of these problems, and in those few cases, the side effects disappeared when I lowered the dosage.

One warning, however. If you're taking a blood-thinning medication such as Coumadin® or aspirin, be sure to notify your doctor. These medications, like ginkgo, have a blood-thinning effect—and the cumulative doses might be more than you need. Your doctor can monitor how well your blood is clotting through regular blood work, by taking blood samples and testing them in the lab.

Recommendations for…

• *Attention Deficit Disorder (ADD).* Although I have not seen any studies on ginkgo and Attention Deficit Disorder, I have had parents tell me that it helps their children with concentration and memory with schoolwork. These are specifically children with memory and concentration problems—not hyperactivity.

• *Alzheimer's disease.* Ginkgo has shown to be of benefit in cases of senility and Alzheimer's disease. In fact, it has been approved for the treatment of Alzheimer's disease by the German government. While it's not a cure—none exists—ginkgo has been shown effective in delaying the mental deterioration that often occurs rapidly in the early stage of the disease.

A study done in 1994, involving 40 patients who had early-stage Alzheimer's disease, demonstrated that 240 milligrams of ginkgo biloba extract taken daily for 3 months produced measurable improvements in memory, attention, and mood.

Most of the patients I see do not have Alzheimer's, but they experience a general decline in short-term memory and concentration. Ginkgo is at the top of the list for safe and effective supplements I recommend. Plus, it is not overly expensive—about $12 to $16 per month at the dosage I recommend—so you won't break the bank if you take it regularly.

• *Circulatory diseases.* Ginkgo is one of the best medicines in the world for improving circulation to the hands and feet. For this reason it's an effective treatment for intermittent claudication.

People who have intermittent claudication—which is really a circulatory problem—experience pain and severe cramping in the lower legs, particularly while walking. This condition is particularly prevalent among the elderly. Many clinical studies have shown ginkgo can help alleviate the condition in 3 to 6 months if you take daily dosages of 120 to 160 milligrams.

Ginkgo has also been shown to improve the condition of people who have Raynaud's disease, a condition where the hands or feet instantly turn blue if you just reach for something in the freezer or step outside on a cold day. (For some reason, women are much more likely than men to suffer from this condition.) Again, the problem is circulatory. I have frequently recommended ginkgo—and achieved positive results —when patients were bothered by cold hands and feet.

Finally, people with diabetes are particularly prone to have poor circulation in their extremities. Supplementing with ginkgo is certainly beneficial.

• *Depression.* Ginkgo is an effective natural antidepressant when the depression is related to poor blood flow to the brain. When blood flow improves, more oxygen and nutrients naturally reach the brain cells as well as extremities.

Ginkgo also improves the activity of neurotransmitters, the brain's chemical messengers. A study of elderly patients who took doses of 240 milligrams of ginkgo extract daily showed that many experienced significant improvements in mood after only 4 weeks. The improvements were even more dramatic after 8 weeks of taking the same concentration of extract.

• *High blood pressure.* Ginkgo is one of the main herbs I recommend to patients who have hypertension or high blood pressure. It helps to relax the artery walls, thus reducing pressure within the blood vessels. A typical dosage would be 120 to 180 milligrams daily.

• *Impotence.* Impotence occurs in the vast majority of cases because there's poor circulation to erectile tissue. Instead of recommending Viagra® to patients with impotence problems, I usually start with a prescription of ginkgo biloba (and sometimes some ginseng as well). Ginkgo works very well, is much less expensive, and doesn't have any side effects—unlike Viagra®.

Because ginkgo improves penile blood flow, it provides the physiological basis for an erection. In one study, 50 percent of patients treated for impotence using 60 milligrams of ginkgo per day regained potency.

I generally recommend 180 to 240 milligrams of ginkgo in the treatment of impotence. If ginkgo doesn't help, I'll have the patient tested for the hormones DHEA and testosterone. If these hormones are deficient, I'll recommend they be used in therapeutic dosages.

• *Memory loss.* Even if you don't remember things so well as you used to, the awareness of memory loss is not a signal of oncoming Alzheimer's disease or senility. Memory loss is quite common—and understandable, given the fact that we do tend to lose some memory capacity as we age and that we are quite susceptible to distractions.

"Cerebral vascular insufficiency" is a phrase that's often used to describe poor blood flow to the brain. Often, the problem gets worse as people get older because people gradually experience atherosclerosis—hardening of the arteries—which sharply decreases the efficiency of blood flow. Simply put, when the brain doesn't get enough oxygenated, nourishing blood, we're more likely to have memory loss. (Depression, as noted, can also be related to restricted blood flow.) Given its power to improve blood flow, ginkgo biloba is the treatment of choice. Once the brain cells get the oxygen and blood sugar needed to help them function properly, memory improves. Clinical studies have confirmed that significant change can occur as rapidly as 8 to 12 weeks.

• *Premenstrual syndrome (PMS).* For women who experience cramping, pain, and breast tenderness around the time of their periods, ginkgo may also provide some benefits. I have been surprised to learn that these typical symptoms of PMS might respond to ginkgo. Studies have shown that ginkgo can be helpful in alleviating breast tenderness and fluid retention.

• *Radiation effects.* After the Chernobyl nuclear accident in 1986, Russian scientists tried a wide variety of treatments to help workers and residents who had been exposed to radiation. Researchers discovered that ginkgo helped combat the effects of radiation. It was found to be a potent agent in fighting free-radical damage to the cells, providing the same antioxidant benefits that help protect normal body cells from the effects of rapid aging.

• *Ringing in the ears (tinnitus).* Studies have been done to test the effectiveness of ginkgo in relieving the condition known as tinnitus, which is ringing in the ears. Results have been mixed. I feel it is worth trying if there's the possibility that tinnitus is the result of poor circulation. Sometimes the condition is related to the fact that insufficient blood is reaching the inner ear. In other cases, however, tinnitus occurs when people are exposed to excessive noise—and in those cases, ginkgo doesn't seem to help very much.

Ginkgo can be helpful if you've had acute hearing loss as a result of pressure changes or sound trauma. Even if you don't know the factors that have contributed to loss of hearing, taking this herb might produce some positive effects.

• *Stroke.* Ginkgo is valuable both in the immediate treatment of stroke and in helping stroke victims during the months or years of recovery. One of the keys to the prevention of stroke is keeping the blood thin. Again, the objective is to improve circulation so sufficient blood gets to the brain. New research is also showing that therapeutic doses of antioxidants may be an important treatment for strokes. As I mentioned, ginkgo provides antioxidant activity as well.

Many doctors who are oriented toward holistic medicine—treatment of the whole patient rather than a single "problem"—often recommend ginkgo to people who are particularly susceptible to a stroke. Among those who need to take special care are anyone with a personal or family history of high blood pressure, atherosclerosis, diabetes—particularly if you're a smoker or if you've had a previous stroke. But remember, many doctors prescribe pharmaceutical blood-thinning medications after a stroke, so if you're taking one of these, you need to talk to your doctor and have some blood work done before you start taking ginkgo, too.

• *Vision.* Ginkgo is also useful in the prevention and treatment of macular degeneration and diabetic retinopathy. If left untreated, both conditions can result in blindness. Macular degeneration, often associated with age, is the result of nerve degeneration in the particularly sensitive light-receptor cells of the eye. Diabetic retinopathy is a serious eye disease that can lead to blindness.

Ginkgo has been shown to be helpful in both conditions. I also recommend ginkgo as part of a natural treatment for cataracts.

■

DR. STENGLER'S RECOMMENDATION FOR HEARING LOSS—GINKGO BILOBA

Take 60 to 120 milligrams twice a day of a 24% flavone glycosides standardized extract. This herb increases blood flow, which helps ear tissues receive the oxygen and the nutrients they need for good health.

■

WHAT YOU CAN DO ABOUT MEMORY PROBLEMS

Misplaced documents. Forgotten names. Missed appointments. More than two-thirds of people over sixty-five say that they have trouble recalling old details and absorbing new ones. To some people, memory problems are just part of what used to be called "senility," an unfortunate but natural part of old age. For others, periodic forgetfulness sets off alarm bells: Is this Alzheimer's? Stroke? Dementia?

Poor memory is a problem but not an inevitable part of the aging process. While it's true that nerve cells in the brain do shrink a little with advanced age and that it's harder for them to form connections with one another, most researchers now believe that memory loss is caused mainly by lifestyle factors. Most cases can be prevented or reversed with some simple changes in diet, exercise, and habits.

Many people with memory problems are actually suffering from a malnourished brain. The brain, like the rest of the body, needs to receive its supply of oxygen and nutrients from the blood if it is to function at its best. Chemicals called neurotransmitters, which enable the brain cells to communicate and create memory links, are especially dependent on good nutrition. The brain also needs high doses of nutrients to fight damage from free radicals. Of particular importance are essential fatty acids, which are required for the cell walls of brain cells. These essential fatty acids, particularly DHA, impact memory and concentration in a positive fashion. When the circulation is sluggish and blood is low in "brain food," memory disturbances may well be the result.

Other factors can contribute as well. Several medications, alone or in combination, can cause memory loss, as can underlying illnesses like depression, thyroid problems, and chronic fatigue. Sometimes even allergic reactions to food can impair memory. Poor digestion can be at the root of memory problems, as can a hormone imbalance. In particular, elevated levels of the stress hormone cortisol can impair memory. One must also consider hypoglycemia as a possibility of poor memory. This makes sense, considering that glucose is the primary fuel source for the brain. Systemic candidiasis frequently causes a foggy or poor memory. Also, toxic metals such as lead, mercury, and others can impair mental function and should be chelated out, if they're a problem.

If you try the suggestions here and your problems don't improve within a couple of weeks, see your doctor.

SYMPTOMS...

• *Difficulty recalling details*

CAUTION: If you have trouble recalling the names of close friends and family members, or if your memory problems began after a head injury, see your doctor immediately.

ROOT CAUSES...

• *A poor diet,* especially one that's high in fat and low in nutrients
  • *Free radicals*
  • *Inactivity, both physical and mental*
  • *Medications*
  • *Abuse of alcohol or street drugs*
  • *Underlying disorders,* such as candidiasis, heavy-metal poisoning, depression, dementia, thyroid disorders, and hypoglycemia

• *Nutritional deficiencies* (especially of DHA, vitamin B-12, folic acid)

TREATMENT...

DIET: A good diet is crucial to brain health.

RECOMMENDED FOOD: Eat a wholesome diet of basic, unprocessed foods. Because conventionally grown foods often contain toxins, buy organic whenever possible. If organic food is unavailable or too expensive, wash your food thoroughly before eating.

The antioxidant vitamins A, C, and E will combat damage from free radicals. Fresh fruits and vegetables are among the best sources of antioxidants, so have a couple of servings at every meal. For vitamin E, add wheat germ to salads, cereals, or juices. Nuts and seeds are other good sources of this vital nutrient.

A deficiency of the B-complex vitamins can cause memory problems. Brewer's yeast is a potent source of B vitamins, as are wheat germ, eggs, and spirulina.

To improve circulation, increase energy levels, and detoxify your body, drink a glass of clean water every two waking hours.

Eat plenty of fiber to keep toxins moving through your digestive tract and to prevent them from taking up residence in your body. Whole grains, oats, and raw or lightly cooked vegetables are good sources of fiber that are also nutritionally dense.

Consume fish, such as salmon, mackerel, and other clean fish, three times weekly for their essential fatty acids.

FOOD TO AVOID: Determine whether your memory problems are caused or aggravated by food allergies. You may want to focus on cutting out wheat and dairy, as allergic responses to these items are most likely to lead to memory problems. If your memory improves when a food or foods are removed from your diet and worsens when they are reintroduced, banish those products from your diet.

Drastically reduce your intake of foods that are high in cholesterol or saturated fat. They impede blood flow.

Avoid sugar and processed foods, which add nothing or very little in the way of vitamins or minerals and actually deplete much-needed nutrients from your brain cells.

Alcohol destroys brain cells, causes dehydration, and clouds the mind. Stay away from it.

DR. STENGLER'S RECOMMENDATION FOR POOR MEMORY

Do you have a poor memory? **DR. STENGLER RECOMMENDS THE FOLLOWING SEVEN REMEDIES THAT CAN HELP MAKE IT BETTER...**

1. *Phosphatidylserine.* Take 300 milligrams (mg) daily. This naturally occurring phospholipid improves brain cell communication and memory.

2. *Bacopa (Bacopa monniera).* This nutrient has been shown to improve memory and recall. Take 300 mg daily.

3. *Ginkgo biloba (24 percent).* Take 120 mg two to three times daily. It improves circulation to the brain, improves memory, and has antioxidant benefits.

4. *Vitamin B-12.* Take 800 to 1600 micrograms (mcg) daily. Consider using a sublingual form at 400 mcg. A vitamin B-12 deficiency contributes to poor memory.

5. *Club moss (Huperzia serrata).* Take a product standardized to contain 0.2 mg of huperizine A daily. This compound has been shown to increase acetylcholine levels in the brain and to improve memory in people with Alzheimer's disease.

6. *Essential fatty acids.* Take 1 to 2 tablespoons of flaxseed oil or 2 to 5 grams of fish oil daily. It supplies essential fatty acids for proper brain function.

7. *Acetyl-L-carnitine.* Take 500 mg three times daily. It improves brain cell communication and memory.

■

FREE MEDICINE AND PENNY CURES FROM THE FUTURE

KEEPING UP THE PRESSURE— AMAZING WAY TO REDUCE STRESS

Many people are aware of acupuncture as a treatment to relieve pain. However, acupressure has been used long before acupuncture in China, Japan, and India. Actually, it could be said that most every culture used acupressure to some degree. Simply, it was pushing on "tender" spots to relieve local pain and discomfort. Sometimes, it's what we do naturally—pressing on a sore, aching muscle, for instance. But practitioners in acupressure and acupuncture have identified less obvious, specific points of the body that can contribute to pain relief or healing.

Chinese medicine has relied on acupressure for over 4,000 years. Today, it remains a major treatment at Chinese hospitals. Its popularity has been growing steadily throughout the world.

CHANNELS OF ENERGY...

The traditional Chinese system of medicine focuses on the concept that the life-giving energy called "Qi" (pronounced *chee*) circulates throughout the body in 12 main channels.

Each channel represents a certain organ system—such as kidney, lung, and large intestine. The points that connect to that system are located bilaterally—that is, on both sides of the body. These channels are all interconnected, so they link up to one another.

Along each of the channels, known as meridians, are specific acupressure points that can relieve local pain and inflammation, and also affect pain or tension in other areas of the body. Many of the points can be used to influence the function of internal organs. It is believed that when there is a blockage of Qi circulation in the channels, then disease or illness arises.

To prevent a disease from occurring, or to treat a disease, one must keep the Qi moving. One way to do this is to stimulate the acupressure points where a blockage is occurring. Usually these points are tender to the touch, indicating a blockage. Whether you relieve sore muscles or an internal problem such as digestive upset depends on which points you press. Mental and emotional imbalances can also be helped with acupressure.

CHEMICAL REACTION?...

It is not known exactly how acupressure relieves pain or improves the functioning of internal organs. One theory is that the brain releases certain chemicals that inhibit pain and stimulate the immune system. It is also thought that acupressure relaxes trigger points so muscle tension calms down.

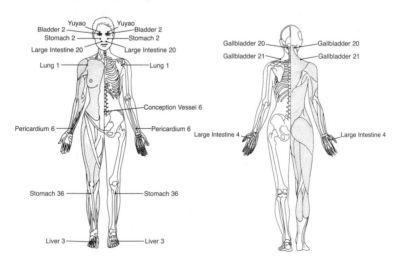

Acupressure may improve blood and lymphatic circulation, as well as improve electrical flow along nerves and between cells. Much research is ongoing in this area, including studies funded by the prestigious National Institutes of Health. Acupressure does work and is a major reason why traditional Chinese medicine is one of the fastest growing medical fields.

While someone trained in acupressure can obtain the best results, there are many easy-to-locate points that you can apply pressure to yourself to alleviate discomfort or improve certain conditions.

ADMINISTERING AN ACUPRESSURE TREATMENT...

Here are four easy steps to follow for self-treatment...

1. *Make sure you are relaxed.* The room should be free of noise. If possible, you should wear light clothing.

2. *Locate the desired point to which you are going to apply pressure.* Press on the point using your thumb or fingers. The pressure should be direct, yet not cause great discomfort. Some points may be very tender, indicating a blockage.

Start with very light pressure, see how you feel, and adjust the pressure accordingly. Press the acupressure point and hold for 10 to 15 seconds. This can be repeated 5 to 10 times to see if it helps relieve the symptoms.

Chronic conditions will need more treatments to see if the acupressure is working. Some people prefer rubbing or massaging the acupressure points; this is fine to do as well. As the same channel runs on both sides of the body, try to stimulate the points on both sides simultaneously. For example, massaging Gallbladder 20 on both sides of the back of the head helps to relax tense neck muscles. Or, Stomach 36, located four finger widths below the kneecap and one finger width toward the outside of the leg (outside the shin bone on the muscle), can be stimulated simultaneously to improve digestive function.

3. *Make sure to breathe while you stimulate the acupressure point.* Slow, deep, relaxed breaths are best.

4. *Relax in a quiet atmosphere after a treatment* and drink a glass of water to help detoxify your body.

WHAT ARE THE SIDE EFFECTS?: Acupressure is a very safe treatment. Temporary soreness of the acupressure point is common and normal. Acupressure should not be applied to open wounds or areas of extreme swelling or inflammation, such as varicose veins.

There are certain points that should not be stimulated on a pregnant woman because of the risk of miscarriage. It is important that pregnant women avoid the use of Gallbladder 21, Large Intestine 4, and Liver 3. Pregnant women should consult with a practitioner of acupressure before self-treating.

Recommendations from the Natural Physician for...

• *Allergies.*

• Large Intestine 4, located between the webbing of the thumb and index finger, relieves nasal symptoms and head congestion.

• Large Intestine 20, located on the lower, outer corner of each nostril, reduces sneezing and nasal symptoms.

• *Anxiety.*

• Pericardium 6, located two-and-one-half finger widths below the wrist crease in the middle of the forearm (palm side), helps relieve anxiety.

• *Cold and flu.*

• Large Intestine 4, located between the webbing of the thumb and index finger, relieves head congestion and sinus discomfort. Gently push on this spot. You want to work this acupressure point on both hands, so after you've treated your left hand, be sure to do the same to the right.

• Large Intestine 20, located on the lower, outer corner of each nostril, reduces sneezing and nasal symptoms.

• *Cough.*

• Lung 1, located in the front of the shoulder area, in the space below where the collarbone and shoulder meet, reduces cough.

• *Constipation.*

• Large Intestine 4, located between the webbing of the thumb and index finger, relieves constipation. Gently push on this spot on both hands.

• *Eyestrain.*

• Stomach 2, located one-half inch below the center of the lower eye ridge (you can feel an indentation), relieves burning, aching, and dry eyes.

• Bladder 2, located on the inner edge of the eyebrows beside the bridge of the nose (you can feel an indentation), relieves red and painful eyes.

• *Headache.*

The following are all helpful. Choose the point or points that provide the most effective relief for you.

• Gallbladder 20, located below the base of the skull, in the space between the two vertical neck muscles.

• Large Intestine 4, located between the webbing of the thumb and index finger. Gently push on this spot on both hands.

• Liver 3, located on top of the foot in the hollow between the big toe and second toe.

• Yuyao, indentation in the middle of the eyebrow (directly straight up from pupil).

• *Indigestion.*

• Stomach 36, located four finger widths below the knee-cap and one finger width toward the outside of the leg (outside of shin bone on the muscle), improves digestive function.

• Conception Vessel 6, located two finger widths below the navel, relieves abdominal pain, gas, and other digestive problems.

• *Muscle pain.*

• Find the points that are most tender in the sore muscle and gently press on them and release, or massage these points.

• *Nausea.*

• Apply pressure on Pericardium 6, which is located two-and-one-half finger widths below the wrist crease in the middle of the inside of your forearm. This point works so well for nausea that special wrist bands can be bought that stimulate this point. They are used for any kind of nausea, including morning sickness and motion sickness.

• Conception Vessel 6, located two finger widths below the navel, relieves nausea and abdominal symptoms. It is also effective for motion sickness.

• *Neck pain.*

• Gallbladder 21, located on the highest point of the shoulder (trapezius muscle), relieves stiff neck and shoulder tension. Feel for a tender spot.

- Gallbladder 20, located below the base of the skull, in the space between the two vertical neck muscles, relieves stiff neck and neck pain.

- Large Intestine 4, located between the webbing of the thumb and index finger, reduces neck and head discomfort. Gently push on this spot on both hands.

- *Sinusitis.*

The following two points relieve sinus pain and promote drainage.

- Large Intestine 20, located on the lower, outer corner of each nostril.

- Large Intestine 4, located between the webbing of the thumb and index finger.

■

THE BUZZ ABOUT APIS

A pis (pronounced *aye-pis*) is a remedy that is derived from the honeybee—the stinger as well as the whole bee. Think of the symptoms that a bee sting causes such as stinging, burning, swelling, and itching. These are all the symptoms for which apis is beneficial. So a homeopathic doctor may recommend it for bee stings, allergic reactions including hives, arthritis, urinary-tract infections, kidney disease, herpes, sore throat, and ovarian pain.

Apis is indicated when symptoms include a lack of thirst, a negative response to heat, and a positive response to cold applications.

Recommendations for...

- *Allergic reactions.* Allergic reactions that cause hives or burning and stinging pains that move around the body can be improved quickly with apis. Apis also improves other symptoms of allergic reaction such as swelling of the throat and eyes. These could be allergic reactions to food or to drugs.

NOTE: Seek emergency medical treatment for allergic reactions, especially if you start to have trouble catching your breath.

- *Arthritis.* If you have swollen joints that burn or sting—and if your joints feel better after applying cold compresses—then the condition can probably be alleviated with apis.

- *Bee stings.* Apis quickly relieves the pain of a bee sting. This is proof of the homeopathic principle that "like cures like." Take it as soon as possible after getting stung to prevent swelling and other symptoms from getting severe. It is a remedy that should be in your home first-aid kit.

- *Herpes.* Apis is a common remedy for herpes infections. Herpes of the mouth—cold sores that sting and burn and that have a vesicle formation—improves quickly with apis. This also applies to the acute treatment of genital herpes.

- *Kidney disease.* Apis is used in acute kidney disease such as glomerulonephritis or nephritic syndrome where there is protein loss in the urine and edema of the body.

- *Meningitis.* Symptoms include a stiff neck, high fever, and dilated pupils. Homeopathic apis is most effective in patients whose symptoms are made worse when heat is applied. This remedy can be used in conjunction with conventional treatment.

- *Ovarian pain.* Apis is specific for right-sided ovarian cysts where there is burning and stinging pain. It not only reduces the pain, but also stimulates dissolving of the cysts.

- *Shingles.* Apis is one of the primary homeopathic medicines for shingles, especially when there is stinging or burning. Apis helps to relieve the pain and heal the shingles.

- *Sore throat.* Apis is very effective for relieving a sore and swollen throat, especially when the sore throat has specific characteristics. Those characteristics include a burning pain (that feels better when you have a cold drink) and a bright red, swollen uvula (the flap of tissue in the middle of the mouth).

- *Toxemia in pregnancy.* Apis is a good remedy for toxemia in pregnancy where there is protein in the urine, high blood pressure, and lots of body swelling.

- *Urinary-tract infections.* Urinary-tract infections can be helped by apis. This is particularly true for bladder infections that cause scalding pain during urination. If you have a right-sided kidney infection, it's another indication that this remedy will probably work well.

DOSAGE: For acute conditions such as a bee sting or allergic reaction, I recommend taking the homeopathic formulation with a 30C potency every 15 minutes for two doses. Then wait and see if the remedy is helping. The other option is to take one dose of a higher potency such as a 200C.

For skin rashes, sore throats, and other conditions that are not so acute, I recommend taking a 6C, 12C, or 30C potency twice daily for three to five days, or as needed for continued improvement.

WHAT ARE THE SIDE EFFECTS?: Side effects are not an issue with apis. It either helps or there is no effect at all. It is also safe to use for children.

■

PLUNDERING THE PINEAPPLE FOR BROMELAIN

Bromelain is actually a group of protein enzymes derived from the pineapple plant, whose healing powers were described in the medical literature as far back as 1876. Though the active enzymes are found in the fruit as well as the stem, commercial products are made exclusively from the stem.

Bromelain is used for many purposes—as a digestive aid, natural blood thinner, anti-inflammatory, mucus-thinning agent, immune-system enhancer, and for skin healing. It also helps improve the absorption of certain supplements (such as glucosamine) and drug medications such as antibiotics.

One of bromelain's unique actions is to reduce inflammation in people who have conditions such as arthritis or heart disease. It can also help control the inflammatory process after an injury. It breaks down blood clots at the site of an injury, so swelling is reduced and, at the same time, there's increased circulation to the site of injury or inflammation. Bromelain also helps control some of the body's naturally produced chemicals that tend to increase an inflammatory reaction after an injury.

MAXING YOUR ANTIBIOTICS...

Bromelain is used in many countries to increase the absorption and utilization of antibiotics.

In one study, 53 hospitalized patients were given bromelain in various combinations with appropriate antibiotic medications. Their conditions included a wide range of health problems, including pneumonia, bronchitis, skin staphylococcus infection, thrombophlebitis, cellulitis, pyelonephritis (kidney infection), and abscesses of the rectum. Twenty-three of the patients had been on antibiotic therapy without success. Bromelain was administered four times a day along with antibiotics or by itself.

To compare, a control group of 56 patients was treated with antibiotics alone.

Of the 23 patients who had been unsuccessfully treated with antibiotics, 22 responded favorably to the combined treatment. The rate of improvement was across-the-board, for every type of disease, when patients were given the combination of bromelain and antibiotics.

For doctors involved in the study, it was an eye-opener. Many had not realized that bromelain was able to potentiate the effects of antibiotics in this way.

I hope we'll see larger-scale studies in the near future. Such promising results suggest that people may be able to take lower doses of antibiotics if they simultaneously take bromelain. (Many doctors are eager to reduce the rampant overuse of antibiotics, which is leading to ominous new strains of resistant bacteria.)

Those with weak or compromised immune systems could be the greatest beneficiaries of combination treatments with bromelain and antibiotics. Infants, seniors, and AIDS patients are particularly good candidates for the combined therapies.

DOSAGE: The dosage of bromelain is designated in two different ways with regard to supplements. One is milk-clotting units (M.C.U.) and the other is gelatin-dissolving units (G.D.U.). Look for products that are standardized to 2,000 M.C.U. per 1,000 milligrams, or 1,200 G.D.U. per 1,000 milligrams. Most people require a dosage of 500 milligrams three times daily between meals.

WHAT ARE THE SIDE EFFECTS?: Side effects are rare with bromelain. However, allergic reactions can occur in sensitive individuals. Increased heart rate and palpitations have been observed in some people at dosages near 2,000 milligrams. Those on blood-thinning medications should check with their doctor first before using bromelain.

Recommendations for...

• *Arthritis.* Bromelain is a popular component of natural arthritis formulas. It is helpful for both osteoarthritis and rheumatoid arthritis.

One study found that the supplementation of bromelain enabled people with rheumatoid arthritis to reduce their corticosteroid medications. In addition, patients noticed significant improvements in joint mobility and also noticed less swelling. This study is encouraging because many people suffer side effects from corticosteroid therapy—and the less medicine they have to use, the better. If bromelain supplementation can reduce the amount of steroids needed, the risk of serious side effects decreases as well.

My experience is that most people with arthritis can maintain a good quality of life if they take the opportunity to try bromelain and other natural treatments.

• *Burns.* A specially prepared bromelain cream has been shown to eliminate burn debris and speed up the healing of burned skin.

• *Cancer.* Various studies have looked at a link between bromelain treatments and cancer deterrence or recovery. In one study, 12 patients with ovarian and breast tumors were given 600 milligrams of bromelain daily for at least 6 months. (Some treatments continued for several years.) Resolution of cancerous masses and a decrease in metastasis was reported.

Bromelain in doses of over 1,000 milligrams daily have been given in combination with chemotherapy drugs such as 5-FU and vincristine, with some reports of tumor regression.

Although I do not rate bromelain as one of the more potent anti-cancer herbs, it is worthy of more study. For those who are using chemotherapy to fight cancer, the addition of bromelain offers the promise of making the therapy more effective.

• *Cardiovascular disease.* Holistic practitioners have expressed a great deal of interest in using bromelain for treatment and prevention of cardiovascular disease. We know that bromelain helps break down fibrinous plaques in the arteries, allowing for more efficient circulation. In theory, at least, this is a sure way to help prevent strokes.

When we take routine tests to determine whether people are at risk of cardiovascular disease, fibrin is one of the markers that we're beginning to look at routinely. (In other words, a lot of fibrin in the blood is one indicator that stroke could be somewhere on the horizon.) The fact that bromelain can help "break down" this fibrin is significant. In one study, bromelain administered at a dosage of 400 to 1,000 milligrams per day to 14 patients with angina (chest pain) resulted in the disappearance of symptoms in all patients within 4 to 90 days.

Bromelain also has the potential to break down plaque, the fatty deposits that impair blood flow through the arteries. The enzyme has been shown to dissolve arteriosclerotic plaque in rabbit heart arteries. While more studies need to be done, I've talked to many practitioners who notice that their heart patients do better on bromelain.

• *Digestive problems.* Bromelain has long been used as a digestive aid in the breakdown of protein, and there are now many "digestive-enzyme formulas" that routinely include bromelain as one of the key ingredients. Either bromelain alone or the enzyme formulas can be helpful for people who have digestive conditions such as colitis or irritable bowel syndrome (IBS). In addition, we know that incomplete protein breakdown is implicated in immune reactions that lead to inflammatory conditions such as arthritis.

• *Injuries.* Bromelain's most well-known use is in the treatment of injuries, and it definitely helps to reduce pain and swelling if you have bruises. In one early clinical trial, doctors gave bromelain to 74 boxers who regularly suffered bruising on the face, lips, ears, chest, and arms. When bromelain was given four times a day, all signs of bruising disappeared by the fourth day among 58 of the boxers.

A control group, comprised of 72 boxers, were given a placebo—a look-alike capsule made up of inert substances. In that group, 62 of the boxers needed 7 to 14 days before the bruises cleared up. (Only 10 were free from signs of bruising after 4 days.)

• *Respiratory mucus.* Bromelain thins mucus. If you have bronchitis and another kind of respiratory-tract condition, you'll probably discover that dosing with bromelain will help you expel the mucus more easily. For similar reasons, taking bromelain has been shown to improve cases of sinusitis.

• *Surgery recovery.* Bromelain is a valuable supplement in helping people recover more quickly from surgery.

In one study, patients who were given bromelain supplements two to four days before surgery were able to recover from pain and inflammation more quickly than those who didn't take the enzyme. The bromelain-takers took an average of 1.5 days to be pain free, compared with an average of 3.5 days for those who went without it. Without bromelain, it took an average of 6.9 days for inflammation to go down, but only about 2 days for those who had bromelain supplements.

In my opinion, supplements such as bromelain should be routinely given to those recovering from surgery. Just think of all the days of suffering patients could avoid!

• *Thrombophlebitis.* In studies, bromelain has been proven very effective in the treatment of vein clots, as thrombophlebitis is commonly called.

• *Varicose veins.* Bromelain has value in the treatment of varicose veins. I do not rate it so effective as horse chestnut and some of the other herbs, but it certainly helps.

■

THE BENEFITS OF MOVING
AND SHAKING—EXERCISE

I wrote this section after coming back from a 3-mile run. I felt great—and knew why. Every time anyone does exercise like this, there's a surge in endorphins and enkephalins—the body chemicals that make you feel good. I was highly motivated to discuss this major component of health and vitality.

Exercise is essentially some form of movement. This ranges from walking to jogging, from biking to playing tennis, to dancing and tai chi, and all the other forms of movement you can think of.

Many people think of a gym when they hear the word "exercise." For some people this brings up images of large muscular men or women grunting and groaning as they lift weights. They equate "exercise" with painful exertion.

My goal here is to get you motivated to exercise and then to select exercises that excite you. I also want you to realize the benefits of exercise and what it can do for you physically and mentally. In addition, I want to give you a sense of what kind of exercise you may want to be doing.

GETTING STARTED...

The first step to a successful exercise program is to get motivated. Think of the health improvements you can get by exercising. Also, think how the quality of your life will improve when you lose weight, gain muscle, and have an abundance of energy.

With more exercise, many areas of your life can improve, including relationships and work. Exercise is also an effective way to increase sex drive and libido naturally in men and women.

Next, think about what will happen if you don't exercise. See yourself as out of shape, having less energy, and your body "falling apart." It's not a pleasant sight. Make up your mind right now that you will begin to figure out and implement an exercise program immediately. Feel good about it and get excited.

I think it's a mistake to select an exercise that you don't really like. For example, a friend invites you to go jogging, so you go, but you really have no interest in jogging. You would rather go swimming. If you pick an exercise that you don't have an interest in, you are not likely to stick with it. For an exercise program to be worthwhile, you have to stick with it over the long term. Studies show that if you abruptly stop exercising, you lose within a couple of weeks most of the benefits that you gained.

Besides motivation, compliance is everything when it comes to getting the benefits of exercise and sticking to an exercise program long term. By choosing one or two forms of exercise that you really enjoy, you increase your chances of sticking with it. Exercise should be something to which you look forward. It's something from which you can gain energy.

CHOOSING THE MIX...

When choosing your exercise program, focus on aerobic work first. By this I mean walking, jogging, biking, swimming, tennis, dancing—any activity that keeps you constantly moving.

By contrast, there is also anaerobic exercise—such as weightlifting—but it's secondary. For example, weightlifting can improve muscular strength, muscle mass, and bone density. It is also good for the heart and cardiovascular system. However, I recommend beginning with an aerobic exercise program, and then adding an anaerobic exercise like weightlifting.

A combination of cardiovascular training like walking or swimming (or many others) plus some form of resistance training like weights is best. This works all the systems of the body.

Don't feel you have to engage in vigorous physical activity to get the benefits of exercise. A study of more than 72,000 female nurses found that women who walk briskly five or more hours a week cut their risk of heart attack by 50 percent.

FREQUENCY AND LENGTH OF EXERCISE...

The frequency and length of exercise depends on your current level of health. Your doctor and a fitness trainer can best determine this. In general, moderately healthy people should start with 10 to 15 minutes of aerobic exercise three times a week and work up from there.

Over time, the length of the exercise period can be increased to 30 to 45 minutes, and the frequency should be four to six times a week. If you experience muscle soreness, and it does not seem to be going away, then cut down the frequency and length of your exercise. If you're starting a weightlifting program, be sure to work with a personal trainer.

If you want some guidance in starting an exercise program, I recommend *Weight Training for Dummies* by Liz Neporent, Suzanne Schlosberg and Shirley J. Archer, and *The Aerobics Program for Total Well-Being* by Kenneth H. Cooper.

WHAT ARE THE SIDE EFFECTS?: Initially, muscle soreness will be the most common side effect as your body becomes accustomed to the exercise. This soreness will become less of a problem after the first three weeks. Proper form is required for weightlifting; otherwise, injuries can occur. In addition, proper warm-up and post-exercise stretching are important to prevent soreness and injuries.

Recommendations for...

• *Anxiety and depression.* Exercise reduces the effects of stress on the body and should be an important part of a treatment program for anyone with these conditions. It also stimulates the release of chemicals in the brain that are important for mood.

A study reported in the *Journal of Epidemiology* showed that those who participated in exercise, sports, and physical activity experienced a decrease in depression, anxiety, and malaise.

• *Arthritis.* The right kind of exercise can be helpful for the different forms of arthritis. For example, swimming is a good choice of exercise for someone with rheumatoid arthritis or osteoarthritis as it is gentle on the joints. Exercises performed improperly, such as running on a hard surface or using an improper weightlifting technique, can aggravate arthritis.

• *Detoxification.* Regular exercise is helpful for anyone in a detoxification program. It promotes increased circulation and lymphatic drainage. It also causes sweating, and thus stimulates detoxification.

• *Diabetes.* Exercise increases insulin activity, reduces total cholesterol and triglycerides, and increases the good HDL cholesterol in those who have diabetes. It also stimulates blood flow that is more easily impeded in someone with this condition. However, anyone who has diabetes should be monitored by his or her doctor, and follow an exercise program under medical supervision.

• *Fatigue.* By expending energy, you can actually increase your energy and vitality level. This is the paradox of exercise, which works well to increase energy levels when done within the parameters of a person's exercise limits. On the other hand, over-exercise can lead to fatigue.

• *Heart disease.* It is a well-known fact that exercise reduces the risk of most cardiovascular diseases. Part of this effect comes from the lowering of cholesterol and triglycerides, and the increase in good HDL cholesterol. It also helps to reduce the effects of stress, another big risk factor for heart disease. Exercise also strengthens the heart muscle. However, anyone who has heart disease should be monitored by his or her doctor, and follow an exercise program under medical supervision.

• *Hot flashes.* Regular exercise has been shown to reduce the number of hot flashes that women experience during menopause.

- *Immunity.* Exercise done in moderation strengthens the immune system. For example, breast-cancer risk is reduced in women who exercise. But it's important to note that over-training, as seen sometimes in marathon runners or triath-letes, for example, can lead to suppression of the immune system. Again, balanced exercise is the key.

- *Osteoporosis.* It is undisputed that weight-bearing exercise stimulates the growth of bone cells and thus increases bone density. Actually, swimming and some other forms of less weight-bearing exercise have also proven to be effective. This is why exercise is so important to prevent and help treat osteoporosis.

- *PMS.* Regular exercise is quite helpful for women who consistently suffer from premenstrual syndrome.

- *Stress.* Exercise is one of the most effective techniques to alleviate the effects of stress on the body and mind.

GINGERROOT—NOT JUST FOR COOKIES

For centuries, ginger (*Zingiber officinale*) has been widely valued as a medicinal herb. It is one of the most widely pre-scribed herbs by practitioners of Ayurvedic and Chinese tradi-tional medicines. The botanical name for ginger is "zingiber," which, in Sanskrit, means "shaped like a horn." Technically speaking, the root is actually a rhizome, a stem that runs underneath the surface of the ground.

It's most commonly used to treat digestive disorders and arthritis in all the healing traditions. It is known as a warming herb, especially suited to people with "cold constitutions," and it's said to enhance circulation. Chinese herbalists use fresh ginger to "warm the lung and stomach."

Ginger is prescribed in Chinese medicine for the common cold, flu, coughs, vomiting, nausea and general digestive upset, and bleeding. It also reduces the toxicity of other herbs, so it's essentially an antidote to plants that might have side effects.

Also, ginger can help protect an intestinal tract that has been ravaged by tainted or toxic food.

To practitioners of traditional Chinese medicine, every form of gingerroot has certain distinct properties. Fresh ginger has a warming effect on the exterior of the body, while the dried ginger is apt to be recommended for warming the middle of the body.

One of the more intriguing Chinese medicine cures is quick-fried ginger, which is made by frying ginger until the surface is slightly blackened. Practitioners say this is the type that's effective for stopping bleeding and treating conditions that affect the lower abdomen.

Today, ginger is used by herbalists and physicians to treat colds, arthritis, digestive conditions, respiratory-tract infections, headaches, motion sickness, and cardiovascular disease.

As with many herbs, ginger has many different active constituents. Dried gingerroot contains between 1% and 4% volatile oils, which account for the strong taste and aroma. (The volatile oils include bisabolene, zingiberene, and zingiberol.) Two of the pungent principles—gingerol and shogaol—are believed to be responsible for a lot of the medicinal effects.

Ginger also contains proteolytic enzymes that help to digest proteins and reduce inflammation. Many commercial products are standardized to the constituent gingerol.

DIGESTIVE POWER...

Ginger has the unique ability to improve many organs that are involved with digestion. Known as an "aromatic bitter," it tonifies the intestinal muscles and stimulates the digestive organs. It also stimulates secretion of bile from the liver and gallbladder, which helps digest fats. Ginger is also a well-known carminative, meaning that it can reduce gas and bloating.

ANTI-INFLAMMATORY...

Ginger acts as a natural anti-inflammatory by inhibiting the release of prostaglandins and other chemicals in the body that promote inflammation and pain. Unlike nonsteroidal medications such as aspirin, it does not have the potential to damage the stomach, liver, and kidneys. For centuries, people used ginger as an anti-inflammatory without knowing how or why it worked. Modern tests have now proven the herb's anti-inflammatory powers.

CIRCULATION AND CARDIOVASCULAR HEALTH...

Ginger promotes cardiovascular health by making platelets (cells responsible for blood clots) less likely to clump together. This preventive action allows the blood to keep flowing smoothly and helps prevent hardening of the arteries.

Studies have shown that this protective effect is achieved by inhibiting the formation of thromboxanes, substances that promote blood clotting. Other substances in ginger promote the synthesis of prostacyclin, a component that helps prevent platelets from "aggregating" or clumping together.

Animal studies have also shown that ginger improves the pumping ability of the heart.

DOSAGE: Fresh gingerroot can be made into tea. It's also sold in capsules, tablets, and tinctures. I have found all these forms to work with patients and myself.

The tea is relaxing and works well for digestive upset, as do the capsule and tincture forms. For the treatment of inflammatory conditions, I recommend a standardized capsule to get high levels of the active constituents that reduce inflammation.

The typical capsule dosage is 500 milligrams two to four times daily. If you're taking the tincture, I recommend 20 to 30 drops two to three times daily.

WHAT ARE THE SIDE EFFECTS?: Side effects are rare with ginger, though some people (my wife among them!) report heartburn after taking it. In the short term, pregnant women can take ginger for nausea and vomiting related to morning sickness. One to two grams appear to be safe and effective.

Ginger stimulates bile production, so some herbal experts recommend that you should avoid this herb if you have gallstones.

Although I have seen no human studies on drug interactions and ginger, it theoretically may cause a problem with blood-thinning medications such as Coumadin®. So check with your physician before using high doses of ginger if you are on a blood-thinning medication.

One last piece of advice you may not find in many books is that gingerroot by itself may aggravate those who are very warm-blooded. If you are the type of person who gets warm and sweats easily, then long-term use of ginger is not recommended just because it can cause discomfort by making you even warmer.

Recommendations for...

• *Arthritis.* Many herbal medicine experts mention that ginger is effective in treating arthritis, but in day-to-day treatment of patients, I have not found this to be true. Ginger by itself does not usually provide substantial relief. That said, however, it can be helpful to some people as part of a comprehensive herbal formula, such as practitioners of Chinese herbal formulas have created for patients with a "cold constitution."

• *Bloating and flatulence.* Ginger is the remedy par excellence for relieving bloating and flatulence, which is the common result of what I call SAD (Standard American Diet). It reminds me of one lady who came up to me after a talk, looked around to make sure no one else was listening, and asked if there was anything I could recommend for her 36-year-old son who was having trouble with a lot of gas. It turns out this son was newly married, and his mother was worried that his flatulence would cause marital problems.

I recommended she give her son a bottle of ginger capsules to use with meals. Hopefully it rescued the young groom from some embarrassment—or possibly saved the marriage!

• *Cardiovascular disease.* Since ginger is a natural blood thinner, it promotes good circulation and therefore improves cardiovascular health. Animal studies show that it helps with the pumping action of the heart. To me, it is most beneficial as a synergistic herb—one that makes other herbs more effective rather than working by itself.

• *Diarrhea.* There's a specific type of diarrhea, called "cold diarrhea" in Chinese medicine, that ginger seems to help significantly. This is the kind that gives you a case of the chills as well as loose stools. (What's called "hot diarrhea," as you might expect, is the kind where loose stools are accompanied by a feeling of feverishness.)

• *High cholesterol.* In animal studies, ginger has been found to lower cholesterol levels in rats. Unfortunately, it doesn't show exactly the same effect in humans. But if you're taking ginger for other conditions, there is a possibility that it could also help lower your cholesterol.

• *Morning sickness.* Ginger has actually been studied as a relief for severe morning sickness. In 19 of the 27 women who took ginger for nausea and vomiting, both symptoms became less frequent within four days of treatment. The dosage of gingerroot capsules was 250 milligrams taken 4 times daily.

Since publication of the earliest studies, which were done in 1990, many conventional doctors have started to recommend gingerroot for morning sickness. (My wife's obstetrician, for instance, recommends it to her patients.) However, I don't advise that women take more than one gram daily during pregnancy, and there's no reason to continue taking it after the morning sickness passes.

• *Motion sickness.* Ginger has received a lot of attention for its ability to prevent and treat motion sickness. A study in 1982 revealed that ginger was superior to the drug Dramamine® for reducing motion sickness. Not every study, since then, has supported this finding, but some excellent research done in 1994—involving 1,741 people—confirmed that ginger was indeed very effective in treating motion sickness.

The 1994 study was done with a group of people who were taking a whale-watching trip. Before boarding the boat, people were asked to take various kinds of motion-sickness remedies, ginger among them. (None of the passengers knew which remedy they were being given.) The study showed that 250 milligrams of ginger was just as powerful as the pharmaceutical medications, but without side effects such as drowsiness.

• *Nausea and vomiting.* Bad food, flu, chemotherapy, and surgical treatments are just a few of the possible causes of nausea and vomiting. No matter what the cause, however, ginger has been shown to be an effective remedy.

In two studies, ginger helped reduce nausea and vomiting in patients who had just undergone surgery where they received anesthesia. (Anesthesia makes some people very nauseated.) If you are scheduled to have surgery, talk with your surgeon about taking one gram of ginger before and after surgery.

■

THE ALL-PURPOSE REMEDY—LICORICE ROOT

In my experience, licorice root is the most versatile of all the herbs. Native to both Asia and the Mediterranean, it has been used by practitioners of Ayurvedic and Chinese medicine for over 5,000 years.

In fact, close to 50 percent of all Chinese herbal formulas contain licorice root. The ancient Chinese texts say it can suppress coughs and moisten the lungs, relieve spasms, and soothe the digestive tract. It is also called a "harmonizing" herb. This means that it helps other herbs to work more effectively to reduce their toxicity when used in a formula.

Licorice also helps detoxify the liver, supports the adrenal glands (your body's major guardians against stress), balances the hormones, and has powerful anti-inflammatory effects.

IMMUNITY BOOSTER...

Licorice contains two substances, glycyrrhizin (pronounced *gle-sir-heh-zin*) and glycyrrhetinic (pronounced *gle-sir-heh-ti-nic*) acid, that have been shown in animal studies to increase the body's supply of one of nature's most powerful antiviral agents—interferon. Interferon helps to keep viruses from reproducing and stimulates the activity of other beneficial immune cells, as well. That's probably why licorice root is found in so many Western, Chinese, Japanese, and Ayurvedic formulas for treating infectious disease.

Licorice root is highly regarded among European physicians as one of the top herbal medicines for combating viral hepatitis. They use the intravenous form for the treatment of both Hepatitis B and C.

DELICIOUS DETOXIFIER...

The Chinese have found through many centuries of using licorice that it reduces the toxicity of other herbs, so they add it to many of their remedies. For example, traditional Chinese herbal formulas containing Ma Huang (containing the chemical ephedrine, which helps open respiratory passageways but can also cause stimulant effects, such as fast heartbeat, sweating, and anxiety), almost always contain licorice root, which helps to prevent these unwanted side effects.

NOTE: The Chinese species of licorice root is *Glycyrrhiza uralensis.* I find it works very similar in action to the kind used in North America—*Glycyrrhiza glabra.*

DOSAGE: For most conditions, I recommend taking licorice in tincture, capsule, or tablet form. As a tincture, take 10 to 30 drops two to three times daily. As a capsule, take 1,000 to 3,000 milligrams daily.

DGL extract comes in tablet form. Chew one or two tablets (380 milligrams per tablet) 20 minutes before meals or take between meals.

WHAT ARE THE SIDE EFFECTS?: High dosages of licorice root (3,000 milligrams daily of the powdered extract or more than 100 milligrams of the constituent glycyrrhizin) taken over many days can have effects similar to those associated with the hormone aldosterone. These include sodium and water retention, and potassium loss, which can lead to high blood pressure. We saw this problem occur when practitioners began recommending very high dosages of licorice root for adrenal burnout and chronic fatigue (which it can help).

Overall, I feel the risk of developing high blood pressure from using licorice is greatly exaggerated. Historically, herbalists have used this root in formulas for thousands of years. The trick is to use it in small amounts.

I do hear the occasional story of someone who feels that taking small amounts of licorice root has caused an increase in his or her blood pressure. This is perfectly possible for people who are very sensitive to licorice root or are low in potassium. As a matter of fact, anyone concerned about high blood pressure should increase his or her intake of potassium-rich foods (bananas, orange juice, vegetables, etc.) and decrease the intake of sodium-containing foods (table salt, canned foods, and restaurant foods). Using table-salt substitutes, which usually contain potassium, can help reduce sodium intake. Multivitamins also contain potassium.

Unless instructed to do so by a natural health-care practitioner, people who have kidney failure and hypokalemia (low potassium blood levels) should avoid using licorice root. Likewise, pregnant women and people with high blood pressure should use it with caution and under medical supervision. Whole licorice extract should not be combined with digitalis and diuretic medications. Taking only the DGL extract (for ulcers) eliminates most of the potential risk for high blood pressure.

Recommendations for...

• *Coughs.* Licorice is an excellent herb to use for coughs, both wet and dry. Licorice has a moistening and soothing effect for dry coughs. It also has a direct cough suppressant effect and is a common ingredient in throat lozenges.

- **Detoxification.** Licorice is one of the herbs to consider when undergoing a detoxification program. As I mentioned, it helps support the liver and should be considered along with herbs like milk thistle and dandelion root. It also works to heal a damaged digestive tract, which is key to long-term detoxification success.

- **Eczema and psoriasis.** Creams containing glycyrrhetinic acid are used to treat inflammatory skin conditions such as eczema and psoriasis. Its effect is similar to that of topical cortisone, and some studies have found it more effective. However, I do not recommend topical treatments (whether natural or pharmaceutical) as the main therapy for skin conditions, as they can simply mask a symptom without treating its underlying cause (e.g., food sensitivities, poor digestion, nutritional deficiencies, etc.). Topical treatments are fine, so long as you also address the internal imbalances that are creating the symptom.

- **Fatigue.** People who experience high levels of stress for long periods of time can suddenly find that their adrenal glands can no longer produce balanced levels of stress hormones, such as DHEA, pregnenolone, and cortisol. As a result, fatigue, poor memory, blood-sugar problems, decreased resistance to illness, and hormonal imbalance can occur.

Some doctors immediately recommend using hormone replacement, and in some cases this is necessary. However, it is worth trying a gentler approach, using supplements such as licorice root, especially to balance out cortisol levels. A typical adult dosage would be 1,000 to 2,000 milligrams of licorice root extract taken daily for two months or longer.

Other supplements that work synergistically to treat this condition include adrenal glandular, ginseng, pantothenic acid, vitamin C, beta carotene, and zinc. In more serious cases, hormones such as DHEA, pregnenolone, and even cortisol may need to be used.

- **Hormone imbalance.** Licorice is one of the better hormone-balancing herbs. It appears to have a balancing effect between estrogen and progesterone, and reduces excess testosterone levels. It is commonly included in formulas for PMS and menopause.

- **Infections.** As mentioned earlier, licorice root is very good for the immune system. The soothing and anti-inflammatory effect of licorice makes it especially good for respiratory tract infections.

• *Inflammation.* Licorice has potent anti-inflammatory properties. Glycyrrhizin is an important constituent that improves the effects of cortisol in the body (powerful anti-inflammatory and antiallergy effects), without the side effects seen with pharmaceutical anti-inflammatory agents such as prednisone. It also inhibits the formation of prostaglandins, which are substances in the body that cause inflammation.

• *Inflammatory bowel disease.* Licorice root is often included in formulas designed to heal conditions such as Crohn's disease and ulcerative colitis.

• *Mouth sores.* Mouth sores, also called aphthous ulcers, can be helped by licorice root. One study of 20 people found that a DGL mouthwash improved the symptoms of 15 of the participants by 50% to 75% within 1 day, and complete healing of the sores within 3 days.

• *Ulcers.* One of the most popular uses of licorice extract is for ulcers of the digestive tract. The recommended form is DGL. It has an interesting mechanism of action: It stimulates cell growth of the stomach and intestinal linings, increases the natural mucous lining of the stomach, increases blood flow to the damaged tissues, and decreases muscle spasms.

In a single-blind study of 100 people with peptic ulcers, participants took either DGL (760 milligrams three times daily) or the medication Tagamet® (cimetidine). Both groups showed equally significant healing of ulcers after 6 and 12 weeks, demonstrating that DGL is as effective as pharmaceutical medications for this condition. Another study of 874 people also demonstrated that DGL was as effective as antacids and the antiulcer drug cimetidine in persons with duodenal ulcers.

More important, DGL actually works to heal ulcerated tissues instead of simply suppressing stomach acid in the way antacids and drug medications do. Remember, with insufficient stomach acid, you cannot digest proteins, minerals, and other nutrients very efficiently. Stomach acid also acts as a natural barrier that keeps bacteria, parasites, and other microbes from penetrating the digestive tract.

■

PASSIONFLOWER FOR INSOMNIA

A climbing vine that can grow upwards of 28 feet, passion-flower grows wild in the southern United States as well as South America. It's also found in the East Indies and in parts of Europe. Historically, Native Americans ate the leaves and fruit of the passionflower and used various parts of the plant to cure ailments. Today, all parts of the plant—root, leaf, stem, and fruit—are used medicinally, although it's mainly the flower parts that are included in capsules, teas, and tinctures.

Researchers believe that certain flavonoids are responsible for the nerve-relaxing properties of passionflower, although other constituents are likely involved as well.

DOSAGE: I recommend 500 milligrams of the capsule form, or 20 to 30 drops (0.5 milliliter) of the tincture form, or one cup of the tea, taken two to three times daily.

WHAT ARE THE SIDE EFFECTS?: I have not read any reports of side effects to passionflower, nor have my patients shown any sign of them. As with any herb, I do not recommend large dosages for pregnant women.

Recommendations for...

• *Anxiety and stress.* Passionflower is an excellent herb for anxiety and general stress. It helps to relax the nerves and muscles without any kind of sedating effect, so it's particularly effective if you want to take something during daytime hours to reduce the effects of stress and anxiety. Passionflower also helps to relax tight muscles.

• *Heart palpitations.* This herb is commonly included in European formulas for treatment of heart palpitations, particularly when there's an underlying component of anxiety. It is often combined with hawthorn berry extract, which is used as a heart tonic.

• *High blood pressure.* I like to use passionflower or valerian in herbal hypertension formulas when stress and anxiety are at the core of a high blood-pressure problem.

• *Insomnia.* Passionflower is particularly good for insomnia related to anxiety. People who experience side effects from sleep medications and even from valerian, have no such problems when they take passionflower.

Passionflower does not cause the drowsiness associated with over-the-counter or prescription sleep medications.

If you are taking it primarily as a sleep aid, I recommend 30 drops of the tincture or 500 to 1,000 milligrams of the capsule form be taken a half hour before bedtime. It is commonly found in formulas that contain nerve-relaxing herbs such as kava, hops, chamomile, and valerian.

• *PMS and menopause.* Passionflower is sometimes used to help reduce the anxiety and irritability experienced by women who have premenstrual syndrome (PMS). We commonly recommend it for the relief of PMS symptoms in a formula that also contains hormone-balancing herbs such as vitex. It is also effective for relief of some menopause-related problems, such as irritability, depression, and insomnia.

RHUS TOXICODENDRON—A SOOTHER FOR ARTHRITIS AND SHINGLES

Rhus toxicodendron (pronounced *roos tox-ih-ko-den-dron*) is the homeopathic dilution of poison oak. We know this as a plant that causes a nasty, blistering rash. However, this homeopathic is one of the best skin remedies for relieving symptoms in people who have touched poison ivy. It is also effective in treating eczema, where the skin is very itchy and feels better after the application of very hot water.

I have also used this for people with shingles. The itching, burning pain of the shingles blisters can be relieved in a few days with rhus tox.

DOSAGE: The typical dosage for rhus tox is 30C potency taken two to three times daily for a day or two for conditions such as stiffness from overexertion. For long-term use for eczema or arthritis, I generally start with a lower dose such as 6C taken two to three times daily.

WHAT ARE THE SIDE EFFECTS?: While rhus tox has few side effects, some people may experience skin irritation. People with chronic eczema or arthritis may experience a flare-up of their condition at the beginning of treatment. This is usually a sign that the remedy is working (known as a healing aggravation).

If you do have a flare-up and you begin taking the rhus tox less frequently, you'll probably notice that the flare-up subsides. Soon after, you'll probably notice an improvement in your condition.

If you are not sure whether you should use rhus tox, consult a homeopathic practitioner.

Recommendations for...

• *Arthritis.* Rhus tox is commonly used for osteoarthritis and rheumatoid arthritis. This is probably the right remedy for you if you notice certain characteristics about your symptoms—they are worse in the morning, improve with motion and activity during the day, and then get worse again at night while in bed.

Rhus tox is also a good remedy if these arthritic symptoms flare up before a storm or in damp weather. It's probably the right remedy for you if hot baths and showers also provide joint pain relief.

• *Flu.* Rhus tox is a good remedy for the type of flu that makes your joints and muscles stiff.

• *Herpes.* Cold sores on the mouth or face, or genital herpes outbreaks can be helped greatly with rhus tox.

• *Shingles.* This dormant chicken-pox virus erupts when the immune system is weakened. Many elderly people suffer from excruciating pain that is often not relieved with conventional medicines. Rhus tox has worked wonders in several cases I have treated.

• *Strains.* Rhus tox should be used when ligaments and tendons are strained. It helps speed up the recovery process. Athletes should have a supply of rhus tox available at all times.

• *Urticaria.* Urticaria is a fancy way of saying hives. For hive breakouts that do not require emergency treatment (such as when the throat closes), rhus tox helps to relieve the itching and works to heal the lesions more quickly. It is also effective for relieving itching caused by mosquito bites.

■

SIMPLE, BUT EFFECTIVE—
SCHUSSLER CELL SALTS

There are more than a thousand homeopathic remedies. Each one has its own set of symptoms on which it is used. The Schussler cell salts are a simplified system that complements the other homeopathic remedies. As you will see, they are easy for the public and homeopaths to use. What is more important, they work!

Have you ever taken a mineral like magnesium to help reduce or prevent muscle cramps, and find that it does not help?

You may not be getting the benefit from the magnesium at the cellular level, no matter how much you are taking. In a case like this, I find that taking the cell salt, or the homeopathic form of the deficient mineral, works quickly to alleviate the condition. The cell salt stimulates a biochemical change at the cellular level, which then gives the desired result.

DOSAGE: Cell salts are used like other homeopathic remedies— and as with other homeopathics, they come in pellet, tablet, or liquid form. The most common potency available commercially is 6x.

Cell salts are best taken 10 to 20 minutes before or after you have any drink or meal. For an infant, you can crush a cell salt tablet and place it on the child's tongue. Or you can mix the tablet with an ounce of purified water and place a few drops in the child's mouth using a dropper or teaspoon. Children like the sweet taste of the pellets and tablets.

When you do take cell salts, however, you'll probably want to avoid strong odors, such as the fragrance of eucalyptus or essential oils.

For acute conditions, cell salts should be taken every 15 minutes or 2 hours, depending on the severity of the condition. For chronic conditions, cell salts are usually taken one to three times daily. Since they are of a low potency, they can be used on a long-term basis.

As described below, one type of cell salts—or a combination of them—can be taken to treat a particular symptom or condition. For example, mag phos helps to relieve muscle spasms. If a person is also experiencing nerve pain, then kali phos could be used as well. These different types of cell salts can either be taken at the same time or in alternating doses throughout the day.

There are also some formulas that combine all the cell salts together in one formula. These are commonly known as bioplasma. They may be used preventatively or to recover from various chronic illnesses.

WHAT ARE THE SIDE EFFECTS?: Side effects are not an issue with cell salts. They either help or do nothing at all.

SELECTING THE APPROPRIATE CELL SALT...

A list of various cell salts follows, with the conditions for which each is used.

• *Calcarea (pronounced kalk-ar-ee-uh) fluorica (calc fluor).* This cell salt is involved in the formation of connective tissue, making it important for the skin, ligaments, and tendons. It is also found in bones. **I RECOMMEND IT FOR THE FOLLOWING CONDITIONS...**

- Abnormal spine curvature
- Brittle teeth and sore gums
- Hard nodules of the breast or other tissues
- Hemorrhoids
- Spine that "goes out" easily (including during pregnancy)
- Sprains and strains
- Varicose veins, weak ligaments, tendons, and joints

• *Calcarea phosphorica (calc phos).* This is the main cell salt for bone health. Interestingly, calcium phosphate is an important enzyme required for bone formation. Calc phos helps in bone formation. **I RECOMMEND IT FOR THE FOLLOWING CONDITIONS...**

- Arthritis
- Fractures
- Growing pains
- Osteoporosis
- Teething

• *Calcarea sulphurica (calc sulph).* This cell salt is a wound- and skin-healer. (It is especially recommended when there is a yellow discharge from the skin.) **I RECOMMEND IT FOR THE FOLLOWING CONDITIONS...**

- Abscess
- Acne
- Boils
- Bronchitis
- Post-nasal drip

• *Ferrum phosphoricum (ferrum phos).* This cell salt is homeopathic iron- bound to phosphate. It is required for red blood cell formation and function. **I RECOMMEND IT FOR THE FOLLOWING CONDITIONS...**
> • Anemia treatment and prevention (iron deficiency)
> • Bleeding (acute and chronic)
> • Fever and infection
> • Heavy menstruation

• *Kali (pronounced collie) muriaticum (kali mur).* This cell salt helps to dissolve mucus. **I RECOMMEND IT FOR THE FOLLOWING CONDITIONS...**
> • Fluid in the ears
> • Sore throat (with white mucus being produced)

• *Kali phosphoricum (kali phos).* This is the primary cell salt for nervous tissue, including the brain. **I RECOMMEND IT FOR...**
> • Anxiety and nervousness
> • Depression
> • Fatigue
> • Nerve injury
> • Poor memory and lack of concentration

• *Kali sulphuricum (kali sulph).* This is another remedy for skin and mucous membrane discharges (especially where there is a yellow discharge). **I RECOMMEND IT FOR...**
> • Bronchitis
> • Eczema
> • Psoriasis

• *Magnesia phosphorica (mag phos).* This is the primary cell salt for the muscles—both internal and external. It also has a tonic effect on the nervous system as well. **IT CAN HELP WITH...**
> • Anxiety and nervousness
> • Hyperactivity
> • Menstrual cramps
> • Muscle spasms and cramps
> • Seizures
> • Stomach cramps
> • Toothache

• *Natrum muriaticum (nat mur).* This cell salt regulates water balance within the cells and tissues. **I RECOMMEND IT FOR THE FOLLOWING CONDITIONS...**
> • Cold sores
> • Depression

- Dry skin
- Edema
- Grief
- Hayfever
- Skin rash from sun exposure

• *Natrum phosphoricum (nat phos).* This is the cell salt that is an acid-base balancer of the cells. **I RECOMMEND IT FOR THE FOLLOWING CONDITIONS...**

- Bladder infections
- Heartburn
- Muscle soreness
- Vaginitis

• *Natrum sulphuricum (nat sulph).* This remedy has a balancing effect on the fluids of the body. In addition, it tonifies the liver and digestive tract. **I RECOMMEND IT FOR...**

- Asthma
- Head injury
- Hepatitis
- Newborn jaundice
- Swelling

• *Silica.* This cell salt is found in the connective tissue, skin, glands, and bones. It acts as a tissue cleanser. **I RECOMMEND IT FOR THE FOLLOWING CONDITIONS...**

- Acne
- Asthma
- Boils
- Brittle hair and nails
- Sinusitis

■

A TREASURE FROM DOWN UNDER—
TEA TREE OIL FOR THE SKIN

Tea tree oil (*Melaleuca alternifolia*), also referred to as ti tree oil, or cajeput oil, has become very popular for its antiseptic and healing properties to the skin. This oil comes from the leaves of the Australian *Melaleuca alternifolia* tree, and early settlers in Australia made tea from these leaves—

which explains the origin of its most common name. But even before the arrival of Europeans, Aborigines of the area were well aware of the medicinal benefits of the oils from this tree.

Most of the research on the medicinal effects of tea tree oil has focused on *Melaleuca alternifolia* in the New South Wales area of Australia.

The first scientific investigations of tea tree oil began in Sydney in 1922 when a government chemist noticed the antiseptic effects of tea tree oil. Though the oils were potent, he observed, they were nontoxic and nonirritating. His initial investigations were followed up by numerous studies, especially in the years between 1922 and 1930. The benefits of this oil became so well established that it was included as standard medical issue in the Australian Army during World War II.

ALL STEAMED UP...

Melaleuca alternifolia oil is extracted from the leaves using a steam-distillation process that extracts only the essential oils. There are approximately 100 chemicals in tea tree oil. Two of the key active constituents are terpinen-4-ol and cineole.

A standard for tea tree oil was established in 1985. It requires a minimum content of 30% terpinen-4-ol and less than 15% cineole. Higher quality oils contain 40% to 47% terpinen-4-ol and 2.5% cineole. The balance between these two constituents is important, with a high-quality product having oils high in terpinen-4-ol and low in cineole. The oil has natural anti-inflammatory, analgesic, antiseptic, and healing properties. It destroys bacteria, fungus, and viruses.

Tea tree oil can be used topically for almost any skin condition. Examples include acne, athlete's foot and fungal infections of the skin, boils, bruises, burns, cold sores, cuts, dandruff, insect bites, rashes, lice, and warts.

It can also be used for gingivitis and vaginitis.

DOSAGE: Make sure to get a product that is 100 percent *Melaleuca alternifolia* oil. An organic product is best. Tea tree oil is generally used in one of three ways—topically, oral rinse, or inhaled.

• *Topically.* When used topically, the oil is placed on the skin. The oil itself can be used, or you can use a cream or gel formula. It can also be used in baths.

Do not apply tea tree oil on infants' skin. Do not use tea tree oil near the eyes.

• *Oral rinse.* When using it as an oral rinse, dilute a few drops in water, gargle, and spit out. It can be used for conditions like gingivitis, toothaches or tooth infections, and sore throat.

• *Inhaler.* To inhale it, add a few drops of tea tree oil to a mister or steamer. You can also put a few drops on a tissue and smell it.

NOTE: Tea tree oil also makes a good disinfectant for washing clothes. Look for laundry detergents made with tea tree oil or add 5 to 10 drops in your washing machine with each load of laundry.

WHAT ARE THE SIDE EFFECTS?: Tea tree oil is very safe for topical use. It is generally nonirritating and nontoxic. It has a pH balance that is almost neutral, so it is not caustic. As with any substance, however, some people could be sensitive to tea tree oil; it is not common but it has been reported in the literature. You can test your sensitivity by putting a couple of drops on your skin before going to bed and seeing if an irritation occurs by morning.

Pure undiluted tea tree oil should not be applied to the skin of children or pregnant or lactating women. These people should use a commercial cream or gel.

Recommendations from the Natural Physician for…

• *Acne.* Tea tree oil has become popular as a treatment for acne. It is applied most commonly as a gel or cream. One study showed that a 5% tea tree oil gel extract was comparable to benzoyl peroxide in the treatment of mild to moderate acne. Tea tree oil users experienced fewer side effects (dryness, burning, redness, and itching). Another technique is to dab the oil on the pimples with a cotton swab before bedtime.

• *Athlete's foot and toe fungus.* Fungal infections of the feet (athlete's foot), toes, and toenails (onychomycosis) are very common and can be stubborn to treat. Tea tree oil has become a popular treatment for this problem.

One study compared 100% tea tree oil to the antifungal topical drug clotrimazole for the treatment of toenail fungus for a period of 6 months. Results indicated very similar results with the two treatments.

I usually have patients trim their toenails, wash feet with soap or tea tree soap, and then apply tea tree oil to the infected area. This needs to be repeated on a daily basis for weeks and sometimes months to eradicate the infection. Another technique is to add 10 drops of tea tree oil to 1 quart of warm water. Soak the feet for 10 minutes and then dry the feet thoroughly with a towel and hair dryer. Continue the treatment for at least six weeks.

Tea tree oil can also be used to combat foot odor (bromhidrosis).

• *Cold sores*. Tea tree oil can be dabbed onto the sores at the first signs of an outbreak. This will keep the lesions under control and prevent the infection from spreading.

• *Lice*. Approximately 12 million cases of head-lice infestation are discovered each year, mostly in preschool- and elementary school-aged children. Lice are extremely small parasites that live and feed on skin. For those seeking a natural, nontoxic approach to this irritating condition, try the following:

Mix 1½ teaspoons of tea tree oil and 1½ teaspoons of lavender oil into 4 ounces of olive oil or 4 ounces of your child's shampoo. Massage this mixture into the hair and scalp. Do not rinse. Cover the head with a shower cap until morning and then comb the hair with a fine-tooth comb. Add 5 drops of tea tree oil to the comb before using it to get out the eggs. Rinse hair and then blow dry for 5 to 10 minutes. (This helps to destroy the eggs.) Repeat this procedure for 7 days.

Tea tree oil can also be used in a shampoo to help treat dandruff.

• *Mouth and gum infections*. Tea tree oil is used for mouth and gum infections, including gingivitis and tooth abscess. Use it as a gargle by adding 3 drops of tea tree oil to 1 ounce of warm water. It can also be purchased commercially as a mouthwash. This treatment can also be used daily for bad breath.

• *Skin infections and eruptions*. Tea tree oil is excellent for the topical treatment of skin infections. It has been shown to be effective against many different types of bacteria and fungus, including *Staphylococcus aureus, Candida albicans,* and many others. It can be used in cream or gel form to treat skin infections such as acne, impetigo, and boils.

It also helps to alleviate the infection and inflammation caused by insect bites. Its soothing and anti-inflammatory properties make it helpful for burns and rashes such as eczema.

• *Vaginitis*. Tea tree oil solutions have been shown to be effective for vaginitis caused by *Candida albicans* and trichomonas. This treatment should be done only under a doctor's care.

• *Warts*. Tea tree oil can be applied topically to warts as it has antiviral properties. It is especially useful for plantar warts.

HOW TO ENJOY YOUR VACATION AND STILL STAY SLIM

Counting calories isn't necessary. Calories are a factor in fat reduction. The higher the number of calories from food, the more energy you must expend burning them off. With my system, counting calories becomes obsolete. The real issue is focusing on quality foods in moderate portions.

If you focus on quality foods and the right ratio of the different types of foods, the calorie count will remain at a level where you can lose weight.

• *Eat smaller meals*. Eating smaller, more regular meals throughout the day helps to quell the appetite and level the blood sugar. This is a long-term strategy for fat reduction.

• *Do not skip meals*. I would say 30 percent of all my weight-loss patients tell me on our initial visit they skip breakfast. Never skip a meal. This is a signal to the body to conserve energy and store fat.

If time is an issue, prepare breakfast the night before or make yourself a protein shake by combining 1 scoop of soy or whey protein powder with soy or rice milk and 1 to 2 tablespoons of ground-up flaxseeds. Add some blueberries or another fruit that you like.

This takes a whopping two minutes and supplies you with protein, carbohydrates, good essential fatty acids, and fiber. It will help to level out your blood sugar and prevent fat storage. It will also increase your energy and mental sharpness as opposed to being tired and mentally dull from skipping breakfast.

• *Harness the power of plant foods.* Don't forget the power of plant foods when you're on a fat-reduction diet. Vegetables and some fruits are excellent sources of fiber, which helps to bind fat from foods and expel it in the stool.

Fiber also helps to slow the release of sugar from foods into the bloodstream. This is especially true of soluble fiber—found in oat bran, dried beans, peas, rice bran, barley, and apple skin.

Plant foods are also excellent sources of phytonutrients that aid the body in many ways, including the process of "burning fat"—that is, fat metabolism.

You can get the full spectrum of amino acids from the combination of various plant foods. They are also very important for detoxification. That's significant because proper detoxification removes toxins that cause fat storage and water retention.

• *Watch your water intake.* Drinking an adequate amount of water is critical for weight loss. Dehydration, even at a marginal level, actually causes the body to store water, and water retention is a large factor in weight gain. In addition, water is essential for detoxification.

You should drink at least six to eight 8-ounce glasses of water daily (48 to 64 ounces). Also, avoid those substances that cause dehydration such as caffeine (coffee), salt, and alcohol.

• *Identify your food sensitivities.* One of the ways I expedite the weight-loss process for my patients is to identify their food sensitivities. Different people are sensitive to different foods. Food sensitivities cause water retention and make metabolism and detoxification more sluggish.

Many of my patients who have had food-sensitivity testing report that they lost extra weight by avoiding the foods to which they are sensitive.

■

WAITER, MORE WATER!

As we all probably learned in school, water is composed of two hydrogen molecules and one oxygen molecule. More than half of our total body weight is water, and a newborn is about three-quarters fluids and one-quarter solid, living human matter.

The brain, surprisingly, is the most concentrated reservoir. There, the concentration of water is almost 85 percent.

About two-thirds of the water in our systems comes from those glasses of fluids that we drink. The rest comes from food and from the leftover "disposables" of cellular metabolism.

Our bodies are really the middle of a streambed. While the water is coming in through various pathways, it's exiting in the urine (60%), evaporating from skin (20%), hissing out through the respiratory tract (15%), and departing in stool (5%).

Water is involved in every single biochemical activity in the body and is required as a solvent for many processes. It is an important component of blood (plasma) and fluids inside and outside the cells. All the tissues of the body—including cartilage and skin—are unquenchable water drinkers. The medium of water is a traveling roadshow, where electrolytes move around, enabling the cells to perform their duty as they generate electrical activity. You need water for detoxification, because waste products course their way out of the body through the multitude of aqueducts—veins, arteries, glands, and organs—that pump, feed, and carry fluids from place to place. Throwing in some thermostatic responsibilities, water also provides a means for temperature regulation.

BODY LUBE...

Humans have a thirst mechanism that is activated when our body is becoming low in reserves of water. Researchers have noted that there is often a long delay between the time when your body actually becomes dehydrated and the moment when you experience the sensation of thirst. In other words, by the time you feel thirsty, you're *already* somewhat dehydrated.

There are a number of symptoms of dehydration that you should be aware of. Thirst, naturally, is one—and any time your mouth feels dry or "sticky," you probably need fluids. Dark urine is another sign.

Many people are in a constant, low-grade state of dehydration. They won't faint, nor do they need to be hospitalized. But that low-grade dehydration can sap vitality and contribute to many of the symptoms I've noted.

Of course, there are situations that lead, almost automatically, to dehydration. If you're in a hot climate, exercising heavily, and not drinking very much, your water reserves drop fast.

But excessive sodium intake—eating a lot of salty foods, including heavily processed food products—will draw water out of the tissues. (I am always reminded of the effects of sodium a couple hours after eating sushi with soy sauce, or foods containing lots of sodium.)

THE DEHYDRATORS...

If you drink a lot of beverages containing caffeine—coffee and soda, for instance—you're sure to have some dehydration unless you also drink lots of water. Alcoholic beverages also have a dehydrating effect.

Any medication that's described as a diuretic, or drugs that have diuretic side effects, will require you to compensate for water loss by getting more fluids every day.

Conditions I see that are related to insufficient water intake include headaches, dizziness, heart palpitations, high blood pressure, irritability, cloudy thinking, skin rashes, kidney pain, and fatigue. Other physicians have noted even more conditions associated with dehydration, ranging from colitis and rheumatoid arthritis to obesity, asthma, and allergies.

Of course, while I'm recommending that people drink sufficient water, I'm acutely aware that many are concerned with the quality of their drinking water. Thousands of people suffer from parasites and other infections related to contaminated water each year. Industrial pollutants and chemicals are traceable in many sources of drinking water. Even the chemicals used to purify water—such as chlorine—have in some cases been linked to cancers such as bladder cancer and, possibly, aggravating asthma. Heavy-metal contamination such as lead, mercury, and aluminum are problems as well.

I advise people to invest in a high-quality filtration system or drink tested bottled water. I also recommend having your local water tested.

DOSAGE: Drink at least six to eight 8-ounce glasses of water daily. If you drink coffee, consume one 8-ounce glass of water for every cup of coffee you drink.

If the weather is hot, drink a glass or two before exercising, and have more than eight glasses during the day.

People on detoxification programs often need to increase their water intake to help flush toxins out of the body.

WHAT ARE THE SIDE EFFECTS?: In rare cases, too much water consumption may place stress on your heart or kidneys. If you have kidney or heart disease, consult with your doctor before drinking larger-than-normal amounts of water.

You may feel bloated if you haven't been drinking very much water and then abruptly increase your water intake. The bloating comes from swallowing extra air—but it won't take long for your body to adjust to increased water intake.

Recommendations from the Natural Physician for...

• *Cloudy thinking.* I call this symptom "brain fog," and most people know instantly what I mean. The mind is not clear, and you find it hard to concentrate. I have seen these symptoms improved with increased water consumption.

• *Dizziness.* Unexplained dizziness may be related to dehydration. Water is required for normal blood pressure. When you're dehydrated, your circulation may be poor, which deprives cells of needed nutrients. Dizziness is one outcome.

• *Fatigue.* Unexplained fatigue can be a result of dehydration. Many people notice increased energy when they drink more water.

• *Headaches.* Patients with chronic, low-grade headaches are often dehydrated. It is often described as a fuzzy sensation in the head.

• *Heart palpitations.* Occasionally a patient reports a history of heart palpitations. These episodes may improve or cease completely when water intake increases.

• *High blood pressure.* You'd think that anyone consuming lots of water would be raising their own blood pressure, but the opposite is true. When you're dehydrated, your body tries to compensate by increasing blood pressure. So for anyone with high blood pressure (hypertension), it's important to increase water intake.

• *Irritability.* There are many reasons for irritability, of course, but if you think dehydration might be one possible cause, there's a quick way to find out—just start drinking a lot more water, and see if your mood improves.

• *Kidney pain.* A number of patients experience kidney pain when they are not drinking enough water. Any kind of kidney pain should be taken seriously. But while you should see the doctor and explain your symptoms, it's also advisable to increase your intake of water. It can't do any harm—and that just might turn out to be the explanation of the problem.

• *Skin rashes*. The skin is a major organ of detoxification. If you're not getting enough water in your system to aid detoxification, you can begin to develop skin rashes of many sorts. Increase water consumption, and you'll help expel some of the accumulated toxins in the body. This is the quickest "first aid" I can think of for treatment of skin rashes.

• *Weight gain and edema*. Your body will retain water if you are chronically dehydrated. This condition, called edema, contributes to weight gain as well. Thus, increased water consumption is an important therapy for helping these conditions.

■

THE MANY HELPFUL USES OF ZINC

Zinc is a mineral with many important functions. Found in all the cells of the body, it's known as a cofactor—that is, a substance required for numerous enzymatic reactions, including detoxification.

It is important for the synthesis and activity of many hormones such as thymic hormone, growth hormone, and insulin, as well as testosterone and other sex hormones. It is necessary for proper immune function and wound healing. It is also needed for protein and DNA synthesis.

Zinc is needed for proper vitamin A metabolism. It is involved in bone formation and in taste.

There are several reasons why people may develop zinc deficiencies. Poor dietary intake is one reason. For example, vegetarians may be more prone to zinc deficiency, as zinc in plant foods is not so bioavailable as in animal products.

Other factors come into play such as genetic susceptibility and some problems with absorption. We also know that certain medications, such as ACE inhibitors like captopril, enalapril, and lisinopril that are commonly used to lower blood pressure, can cause zinc deficiency. Other problematic drugs are aspirin and the birth-control pill.

The elderly are more prone to a deficiency because digestive powers decrease as we age, and our bodies don't absorb zinc so well. Alcoholics are at risk for zinc deficiency, and so is anyone with a metabolic disease such as diabetes. When people have diseases of the digestive tract such as Crohn's disease or Celiac disease, and just have general malabsorption—caused by leaky gut syndrome, for instance—they may have impaired mineral absorption.

WHEN ZINC IS MISSING...

Severe nutritional deficiencies are not that common—but I often see people who have marginal or subclinical deficiencies. SYMPTOMS AND CONDITIONS ASSOCIATED WITH ZINC DEFICIENCY INCLUDE THE FOLLOWING...

- *Poor wound healing*
- *Lowered immunity; susceptibility to infections*
- *Poor skin and nail health (nails may have white spots)*
- *Fatigue*
- *Loss of taste and smell*
- *Poor growth and development*
- *Blood sugar imbalance*
- *Anorexia; reduced appetite*
- *Delayed sexual development and maturation*
- *Night blindness (due to involvement with vitamin A metabolism)*
- *Infertility*
- *Skin abnormalities*
- *Dandruff*
- *Impaired nerve conduction*
- *Hair loss*
- *Prostate enlargement*
- *Birth malformations*
- *Psychiatric illness*

GETTING YOUR ZINC...

The recommended daily allowance is 15 milligrams per day for adult males and 12 milligrams for adult females. Good food sources include fish and seafood such as oysters and other shellfish. Red meat is also high in zinc.

Eggs and milk also contain ample amounts of zinc. Plant foods such as whole grains and cereals, legumes, nuts, and seeds (particularly pumpkin seeds) contain good amounts of zinc, but the mineral isn't so bioavailable as the zinc that comes from animal products.

Breast milk contains a good supply of zinc, so infants are well protected.

DOSAGE: Adults can benefit from supplementing with an extra 15 to 30 milligrams daily of zinc. Most high-potency multivitamins contain this amount.

Children under one year of age can use a pediatric multivitamin that contains up to 5 milligrams. Children over the age of one can take a children's multivitamin that contains 5 to 15 milligrams in each daily dose.

For specific conditions, such as wound healing or acne, higher dosages of up to 100 milligrams daily may be required for a limited amount of time.

Avoid the use of zinc sulfate, which is not readily absorbed. I recommend other formulas such as zinc picolinate, zinc monomethionine, zinc citrate, and zinc chelate.

NOTE: If you are taking a calcium supplement, take it at a different time from when you take your zinc supplement. The calcium may hinder zinc absorption.

WHAT ARE THE SIDE EFFECTS?: Zinc is actually quite a safe supplement, though some people may experience digestive upset if they take zinc on an empty stomach.

High dosages of 150 to 200 milligrams or more, taken over a long period of time, might cause depressed immunity. But I don't recommend taking such high doses anyway, even if you're treating a condition such as severe acne.

One concern is the possibility of developing copper anemia if you are taking high dosages of zinc without taking copper. In the absence of copper, red blood cells change shape; when that happens, they don't carry oxygen so efficiently.

Recommendations from the Natural Physician for...

• *Acne.* Zinc is involved in the metabolism of testosterone. As that "male hormone" is metabolized, it is converted to a metabolite hormone known as DHT (dihydrotestosterone). High levels of DHT are associated with the development of acne, because it increases sebum production. Zinc works to reduce the conversion and also promotes skin healing. Many studies have shown that zinc is beneficial for acne treatment, and at least one indicated that zinc is as effective as tetracycline.

• *AIDS*. People with AIDS are prone to several nutritional deficiencies. Zinc is one of the critical minerals for the immune system, therefore an essential supplement if you have AIDS.

• *Alzheimer's disease*. Zinc may be helpful in slowing the progression of Alzheimer's disease. In a study that included ten people who had Alzheimer's, researchers found that supplementation with zinc helped eight of the people improve memory and communication.

• *Atherosclerosis*. Zinc appears to be one of the many nutrients that helps to prevent atherosclerosis.

• *Birth complications*. Zinc is important during pregnancy because it is required for cell division. A deficiency of zinc is linked to conditions such as premature birth, low birth weight, growth retardation, and preeclampsia. A good prenatal multivitamin should help prevent a zinc deficiency when used in combination with a balanced diet.

• *Burns, cuts, and wounds*. Zinc is needed for cell division and protein synthesis, both of which are required for skin and wound healing. Burns, cuts, and other skin traumas can be relieved with zinc supplements. By taking supplements, you can also speed healing.

• *Common cold*. Several studies have shown that zinc lozenges reduce the severity and duration of the common cold, and also help to relieve sore throats that accompany a cold. It is helpful to take zinc lozenges containing 15 to 25 milligrams of elemental zinc at the first signs of a cold. I find they are particularly good for healing a sore throat.

• *Eating disorders*. Zinc is involved in producing stomach acid as well as stimulating a normal appetite. Studies have shown that people with anorexia and bulimia have deficient zinc levels and may benefit from zinc supplements. Holistic practitioners recommend zinc as part of a comprehensive protocol for people with these eating disorders.

• *Macular degeneration*. Zinc is important in maintaining normal vision. One study of 155 people with macular degeneration found that 45 milligrams of zinc per day significantly slowed the rate of visual loss.

The macula is the portion of the eye that is responsible for fine vision, and when there's degeneration in that area, the sight begins to go. In fact, macular degeneration is the leading cause of blindness in the aged. There are two main types—"dry" and "wet." Nutritional therapy is mainly used for the dry type.

I usually recommend combining zinc supplementation with other important supplements including vitamin C, selenium, carotenoids, taurine, lutein, and the herbs ginkgo and bilberry.

• *Male infertility.* Men who are deficient in zinc may have decreased testosterone and sperm production. Studies have shown that zinc supplements increase sperm counts and testosterone in men who previously had deficiencies that prevented conception.

In one study, 11 men who were infertile were treated with 55 milligrams of zinc daily for 6 to 12 months. They showed an increase in sperm count and motility—and three of the men's wives became pregnant during the study.

• *Prostate enlargement.* Zinc is an effective treatment for prostate enlargement. The mineral inhibits the enzyme 5-alpha reductase, which converts testosterone to dihydrotestosterone (DHT). Since high levels of DHT are believed to promote prostate enlargement, I generally prescribe 90 to 100 milligrams daily for men with this condition. After two months, I recommend reducing the zinc dosage to a maintenance level of 50 milligrams.

• *Wilson's disease.* Zinc is one of the primary treatments for this genetic disease in which copper accumulates in the liver and body, causing brain damage. High doses of zinc help to hinder copper absorption.

■

This chapter is excerpted from *The Natural Physician's Healing Therapies* by Mark Stengler, ND. © 2001 Prentice Hall Press. Permission of Penguin USA.

4

HOW TO RESEARCH DIETARY SUPPLEMENTS ON THE WEB

HOW TO CHOOSE THE BEST INTERNET SITES

An easy way to get information about dietary supplements is to look it up on the Internet. Start with the Web sites of organizations, rather than doing blind searches using a search engine. **HERE ARE SOME QUESTIONS TO CONSIDER...**

WHO OPERATES THE SITE?...

Is the site run by the government, a university or a reputable medical or health-related association (such as the American Medical Association, American Diabetes Association, American Heart Association or the National Institutes of Health)? Is the information written or reviewed by qualified health professionals, experts in the field, academia, government or the medical community?

WHAT IS THE PURPOSE OF THE SITE?...

Is the purpose of the site to educate the public objectively or just to sell a product? Be aware of practitioners or organizations whose main interest is in marketing products, either directly or through sites with which they are linked. Commercial sites should clearly distinguish scientific information from advertisements. Most nonprofit and government sites contain no advertising, and access to the site and materials offered are usually free.

WHAT IS THE SOURCE OF THE INFORMATION AND DOES IT HAVE ANY REFERENCES?...

Has the study been reviewed by recognized scientific experts and published in reputable peer-reviewed scientific journals, like *The New England Journal of Medicine*? Does the information say "some studies show..." or does it state where the study is listed so that you can check the authenticity of the references? For example, can the study be found in the National Library of Medicine's database of literature citations (*www.nlm.nih.gov*)?

HOW RECENT IS THE INFORMATION?...

Check the date when the material was posted or updated. Often, more recent research or other findings will not be reflected in older material. For example, side effects or interactions with other products may have just been discovered, but that information won't appear on the Web site. Ideally, health and medical sites should be updated frequently.

Here are some government and nonprofit sources of health and medical information...

• *American Botanical Council,* P.O. Box 144345, Austin, TX 78714. 512-926-4900, *www.herbalgram.org.*

• *American Cancer Society,* 1599 Clifton Road NE, Atlanta, GA 30329. 800-227-2345, *www.cancer.org.*

• *American Heart Association,* 7272 Greenville Avenue, Dallas, TX 75231. 800-242-8721, *www.americanheart.org.*

• *American Medical Association,* 515 N. State Street, Chicago, IL 60610. 800-621-8335, *www.ama-assn.org.*

• *Centers for Disease Control and Prevention,* 1600 Clifton Road, Atlanta, GA 30333. 800-311-3435, *www.cdc.gov.*

• *FirstGov for Consumers, U.S. General Services Administration,* 1800 F Street NW, Washington, DC 20405. 800-333-4636, *www.consumer.gov.*

• *Food and Drug Administration,* 5600 Fishers Lane, Rockville, MD 20857. 888-463-6332, *www.fda.gov.*

- *International Food Information Council,* 1100 Connecticut Avenue NW, Washington, DC 20036. 202-296-6540, *www.ific.org.*

- *MedWatch,* FDA Safety Information and Adverse Event Reporting Program, US Food and Drug Administration, 5600 Fishers Lane, Rockville, MD 20857. 888-463-6332, *www.fda. gov/medwatch/safety.htm.*

- *MayoClinic.com,* 200 First Street SW, Rochester, MN 55905. 507-284-2511, *www.mayoclinic.com.*

- *Memorial Sloan-Kettering Cancer Center,* 1275 York Avenue, New York, NY 10021. 800-525-2225, *www.mskcc.org.*

- *National Cancer Institute,* 6116 Executive Boulevard, Room 3036A, Bethesda, MD 20892. 800-422-6237, *www.cancer.gov.*

- *National Center for Complementary and Alternative Medicine,* National Institutes of Health, 9000 Rockville Pike, Bethesda, MD 20892. 888-644-6226, *http://nccam.nih.gov.*

- *National Institute of Allergy and Infectious Diseases,* 6610 Rockledge Drive, MSC 6612, Bethesda, MD 20892. 301-496-5717, *www.niaid.nih.gov.*

- *National Library of Medicine,* 8600 Rockville Pike, Bethesda, MD 20894. 888-346-3656, *www.nlm.nih.gov.*

Here are other Web sites that offer health information, especially about herbs and supplements...

- *AARP,* 601 E Street NW, Washington, DC 20049. 888-687-2277, *www.aarp.org/health/staying_healthy/eating.*

- *Magaziner Center for Wellness & Anti-Aging Medicine,* 1907 Greentree Road, Cherry Hill NJ 08003. 856-424-8222, *www. drmagaziner.com.*

- *Medical Network,* Windsor Corporate Park, 50 Millstone Road, Building 200, Suite 160, East Windsor, NJ 08520. 609-426-4620, *www.healthatoz.com.*

- *MindBodyFocused,* 5928 Geiger Ct., Carlsbad, CA 92008. 800-549-3904, *www.mindbodyfocused.com/body/nutritional-supplements.php.*

- *NaturalHealthWeb.com,* 20 Arie Drive, Marlboro, NJ 07746. 732-761-9930, *www.naturalhealthweb.com.*

- *WebMD,* 111 Eighth Avenue, 7th floor, New York, NY 10011. 212-624-3700, *www.webmd.com.*

■

WHERE TO BUY SUPPLEMENTS

• *AdvantageNutrition.com*, 8595 Cox Lane, Cutchogue, NY 11935. 800-211-1303, *www.advantagenutrition.com*.

• *Affordable Supplements*, 4105 West Pawnee, Wichita, KS 67209. 877-478-3678, *www.affordablesupplements.com*.

• *AllStarHealth.com*, 16692 Burke Lane, Huntington Beach, CA 92647. 800-875-0448, *www.allstarhealth.com*.

• *Alterna-Med Inc./VitaminProShop.com*, 10703 West 63 Street, Shawnee, KS 66203. 913-631-4777, *www.vitaminproshop.com*.

• *American Nutrition*, 735 North Park Street—Unit E, Castle Rock, CO 80109. 800-454-3724, *www.meganutrition.com*.

• *Drugstore.com*, 411 108th Avenue NE, Suite 1400, Bellevue, WA 18004. 800-378-4786, *www.drugstore.com*.

• *Eclectic Institute*, 36350 SE Industrial Way, Sandy, OR 97055. 800-332-4372, *www.eclecticherb.com*.

• *eVitamins*, 6060 Collection Drive, Suite 101, Shelby Twp., MI 48316. 888-222-6056, *www.evitamins.com*.

• *Freeda Vitamins*, 47-25 34th Street, Third Floor, Long Island City, NY 11101. 800-777-3737, *www.freedavitamins.com*.

• *General Nutrition Centers*, 300 Sixth Avenue, Pittsburgh, PA 15222. 877-462-4700, *www.gnc.com*.

• *Greatest Herbs on Earth*, P.O. Box 60635, Lemmon Valley, NV 89506. 775-996-1327, *www.greatestherbsonearth.com*.

• *Health Catalog*, 460 Oak Street, Suite 104, Glendale, CA 91204. 800-651-0062, *www.healthcatalog.com*.

• *Healthway Natural Foods*, P.O. Box 129, Paeonian Springs, VA 20129. 703-589-1041, *www.healthwaynaturalfoods.com*.

• *Herbal Remedies USA*, 225 N. Wolcott, Casper, WY 82601. 866-467-6444, *www.herbalremedies.com*.

• *Herb Shop*, 49-B Bryant Street, Jasper, GA 30143. 800-760-0733, *www.herbshop.com*.

• *Hilife Vitamin and Herb Co.*, 48 River Road, Chatham, NJ 07928. 800-622-8877, *www.hilife-vitamins.com*.

- *InternationalSupplements.com*, 2776 Ravella Way, Suite 1206, Palm Beach Gardens, FL 33410. 800-476-1720, *www. internationalsupplements.com.*

- *Kosher Vitamins Express*, 5203 13th Avenue, Brooklyn, NY 11219. 800-645-1899, *www.koshervitamins.com.*

- *MedWing.com*, 1082 South Roger Circle, Boca Raton, FL 33487. 877-633-9464, *www.medwing.com.*

- *Mother Nature*, 322 Seventh Avenue, Third Floor, New York, NY 10011. 800-439-5506, *www.mothernature.com.*

- *Natural Connections*, 301 West Harford Street, Milford, PA 18337. 800-297-7341, *www.naturalconnections.com.*

- *NutriCraze.com*, 5715 Will Clayton #1919, Humble, TX 77338. 800-936-1869, *www.nutricraze.com.*

- *RippleCreek.com*, P.O. Box 1165, Southport, CT 06890. 203-331-0363, *www.ripplecreek.com.*

- *Smartbomb.com*, 66 Morris Street, Morristown, NJ 07960. 800-425-3115, *www.smartbomb.com.*

- *Spring Valley Herbs and Natural Foods*, 1738 S. Glenstone, Springfield, MO 65804. 800-967-3982, *www.springvalleyherbs. com.*

- *SuperValueVitamins.com*, 1461 Main Street, Sarasota, FL 34236. 866-966-1900, *www.supervaluevitamins.com.*

- *The Herbs Place*, 27 Fleetwood Drive, Palmyra, VA 22963. 866-580-3226, *www.theherbsplace.com.*

- *Total Health Discount Vitamins*, 120 Broadhollow Road (Route 110), Suite 1, Farmingdale, NY 11735. 800-283-2833, *www.totaldiscountvitamins.com.*

- *VirtuVites*, 735 N. Park Street, Unit E, Castle Rock, CO 80104. 800-332-5069, *www.virtuvites.com.*

- *Vitacost.com*, 2055 High Ridge Road, Boynton Beach, FL 32426. 800-381-0759, *www.vitacost.com.*

- *VitaminBargain.com*, 636 Kinderkamack Road, River Edge, NJ 07661. 201-986-0818, *www.vitaminbargain.com.*

- *Vitamin Connection*, 121 Connor Way, Suite 130, Williston, VT 05495. 800-760-3020, *www.vitamin-connection.com.*

- *Vitamin Express,* 1428 Irving Street, San Francisco, CA 94122. 800-500-0733, *www.vitaminexpress.com.*

- *VitaminLife,* 15940 Redmond Way, Redmond, WA 98052. 866-998-8855, *www.vitaminlife.com.*

- *Vitamin Shoppe,* 2101 91st Street, North Bergen, NJ 07047. 800-223-1216, *www.vitaminshoppe.com.*

- *VNF Nutrition,* 1029-C Route 112, Port Jefferson Station, NY 11776. 800-681-7099, *www.vnfnutrition.com.*

■